NOTES ON NIGHTINGALE

A volume in the series

The Culture and Politics of Health Care Work
edited by Suzanne Gordon and Sioban Nelson

A list of titles in this series is available at www.cornellpress.cornell.edu.

NOTES ON NIGHTINGALE

THE INFLUENCE AND LEGACY OF A NURSING ICON

EDITED BY
SIOBAN NELSON AND ANNE MARIE RAFFERTY

ILR PRESS

AN IMPRINT OF
CORNELL UNIVERSITY PRESS
ITHACA AND LONDON

First published 2010 by Cornell University Press
First printing, Cornell Paperbacks, 2010

Printed in the United States of America

Library of Congress Cataloging-in-Publication Data

Notes on Nightingale : the influence and legacy of a nursing icon / edited by Sioban Nelson and Anne Marie Rafferty.
    p. cm. — (The culture and politics of health care work)
  Includes bibliographical references and index.
  ISBN 978-0-8014-4906-2 (cloth : alk. paper) —
  ISBN 978-0-8014-7611-2 (pbk. : alk. paper)
  1. Nightingale, Florence, 1820–1910—Influence.   2. Nursing—
Philosophy.   I. Nelson, Sioban.   II. Rafferty, Anne Marie.
III. Series: Culture and politics of health care work.

  RT37.N5.N68 2010
  610.73—dc22

                                                    2010002266

Cornell University Press strives to use environmentally responsible suppliers and materials to the fullest extent possible in the publishing of its books. Such materials include vegetable-based, low-VOC inks and acid-free papers that are recycled, totally chlorine-free, or partly composed of nonwood fibers. For further information, visit our website at www.cornellpress.cornell.edu.

Cloth printing   10 9 8 7 6 5 4 3 2 1
Paperback printing   10 9 8 7 6 5 4 3 2

CONTENTS

FOREWORD

For me, as a child, Florence Nightingale was a vivid presence of whom my father and grandfather spoke with respect and admiration. My grandfather had known her well. When he was a child, she often stayed at Claydon House, the family home. Her relationship with him and his siblings was intense and intimate, and his great love and respect for her and for her determination, authority, and spiritual dedication to service was passed down to us.

It is exciting to me to have found just these qualities appreciated in this major contribution to Nightingale scholarship. This book is vibrant with the ideas of its subject and its authors. Florence Nightingale was very much a woman of her class and time, and she thought prayerfully and practically about the very new problems of nineteenth-century society. Despite her uncertain health, she maintained her intellectual energy, passion, and independence into old age.

To assess Florence Nightingale's influence on progressive thinking about the social policy of her time will always be difficult. The new perspectives revealed through this book may prove these ideas to be as widespread and long lasting as the simpler, popular image of the lady with the lamp.

RACHEL VERNEY Visiting Associate, Florence Nightingale School of Nursing and Midwifery, London, August 2009. Ms. Verney's great-great-grandmother was Florence Nightingale's elder sister, (Frances) Parthenope Verney (née Nightingale) (1819–1890).

NOTES ON NIGHTINGALE

INTRODUCTION

SIOBAN NELSON AND ANNE MARIE RAFFERTY

The centenary of the death of Florence Nightingale occurs on 13 August 2010. Like Charles Darwin, Charles Dickens, and John Stuart Mill, Nightingale is one of those monumental Victorians who were genuine household names in their day and for the generations that followed. Like her peers, she was a highly educated individual on a lifelong path of discovery, dedicated to knowledge and science in the service of a better society. But Nightingale was a singular individual among the great Victorians in that she was a woman—a woman who achieved a level of fame arguably surpassed only by the queen herself. Nightingale was also exceptional in that the work for which she is best known was not her science, literature, or philosophy, but the professionalizing of a domain of low status and semidomestic women's work: nursing.

Nightingale is a fascinating figure, a true polymath who engaged in a multitude of intellectual projects throughout her long life. She was a woman of privileged background, well educated and socially connected, who made her mark in a number of critical fields. A prodigious writer and formidable thinker, she was deeply engaged in the major debates concerning social reform and in the intellectual and religious discussions that marked the second half of the nineteenth century. Her long life provides the researcher with a plenitude of sources from her published writings and reports, which she wrote both alone and with collaborators, as well as her prodigious personal correspondence with individuals, organizations, and governments throughout the British Empire and the rest of the world.

Nightingale has also been the subject of an industry in biographies, from mid-nineteenth-century short stories of her life; to the authoritative work of E. T. Cook, which was commissioned on her death by her family and published in 1913; to Mark Bostridge's 2008 magisterial biography, which balances the rich, textured complexity of Nightingale's character against the canvass of challenges she confronted and set herself.[1] This overwhelming amount of scholarship on Nightingale attests to the fact that a century after her death she continues to draw the historian, the biographer, and the nursing scholar alike to explore her life, her thoughts, and her legacy. Best known for her campaign to improve hospital care and her crusade to introduce training for nurses, she is less well known for her public health campaign, principally seeking to influence British policy in India but also at home and around the world. Even less well known are her contributions to the nascent field of statistics (her great passion) and her philosophical and theological writings, which provide enormous insight not only into Nightingale but also into the spiritual and intellectual character of the Victorian era.

Intellectually, Nightingale was greatly influenced by the Sanitary Movement for public health and supported the ideas of Edwin Chadwick, William Farr, and other public health thinkers.[2] Sanitarians believed that disease was caused by miasma, or foul air, and thus the main strategy to improve health was to improve ventilation and to engineer innovations that provided for clean drinking water and the efficient disposal of sewage. The assumption that disease prevention is an environmental and community problem and does not reside within an individual was one that underpinned Nightingale's life's work. When she tackled the hospital from this perspective and focused on the training of nurses as the critical intervention that society needed to bring about improvements in health, her impact was remarkable and her legacy profound.

Who was Nightingale? A quick search of Google or Wikipedia or the BBC online instructional site for school children, or the literally hundreds of other sites maintained by enthusiasts such as nursing organizations, individual nurses, and Country Joe MacDonald, to name a few, provides the basic facts.

Florence Nightingale was born in 1820 in Florence, Italy, the second daughter of influential and wealthy parents, William and Frances (Fanny) Nightingale. Her home education was extensive, and she was a talented scholar, particularly gifted at mathematics. A serious and religious child, Nightingale experienced a call from God to his service. Her interest in helping relatives and members of the local community when sick was followed by an effort to learn every aspect of care of the sick as well as hospital management. Her self-styled program of study led her to visit well-known sites of hospital care such as the famous deaconess hospital at Kaiserswerth in Germany, which was under the directorship of Pastor Theodore Fliedner. She also spent time visiting an array of Catholic hospitals in France and Italy and briefly nursed at a hospital in Paris. In 1853 Nightingale had some opportunity to move from theory to practice when she assumed the role of superintendent of the Establishment for Gentlewomen during Illness at Upper Harley Street.

All this background was preparation for her major life role, leading the nursing mission to the Crimean War (1853–56), in which France, Britain, Ottoman Turkey, and Sardinia-Piedmont fought Russia over control of territories opened up by the decline of the Ottoman Empire. By 1854 the British campaign was floundering as soldiers died in massive numbers from disease (cholera, typhoid, and dysentery). The public became aware of the appalling conditions in the British military hospitals as a result of reports published in *The Times*. Even worse, it was learned that the French were better organized and benefited from the care of religious nurses, the Daughters of Charity. The resulting furor led to Nightingale's invitation by her friend and colleague Sidney Herbert, secretary at war, to lead a delegation of nurses.

The rest, as they say, is history. Nightingale's two-year work in Scutari, Turkey, involved the implementation of sanitarian principles (hygiene, ventilation, light, nourishing diet, and activity) along with advocacy for better resources for the hospitals and for the injured and sick soldiers. Public fascination with this work and her personal high profile brought the question of hospital reform and the training of nurses to the forefront of British consciousness. Within a year of the end of the war in 1856, Nightingale had been immortalized as the "Lady with a Lamp" of Longfellow's poem *Santa Filomena* and was made responsible for the Nightingale Fund of £45,000, which had been established by a grateful public to begin the training of nursing. The war also led to Nightingale's lifelong incapacitation from poor health due to her contraction of "Crimean Fever," what is now thought to have been brucellosis from contaminated milk products.

A reluctant public figure, Nightingale avoided the spotlight and spent a great deal of the remainder of her life confined to her room. Despite this reclusiveness, she was deeply engaged in public life. She authored influential reports on the sanitary conditions in various contexts, such as military hospitals and public health in India. In 1859 she wrote her landmark text, *Notes on Nursing: What It Is and What It Is Not*. This enormously popular book has been in publication (in many languages) since that time.[3] Another recent anniversary, this time the one hundred fiftieth, is that of the nursing school founded by Nightingale under the auspices of the Nightingale Fund. In 1860 Nightingale oversaw the establishment of St. Thomas' School of Nursing, the world's first formal secular training school for nurses. The school, which opened its doors on 9 July to the first probationers,[4] was known as the Nightingale School of Nursing and is still an eponymously named school within King's College, London.

Throughout her life Nightingale remained absorbed in her work. As a formidable researcher and thinker and tireless correspondent, she wielded phenomenal influence on the reform agenda for military hospitals, the development of nursing around the world, sanitation reform in India, and countless other topics. Bedridden for her final decade, she died at the age of ninety and was buried, in accord with her wishes, without fanfare, in a country churchyard near her family home in Hampshire. The *Guardian* obituary described her task in Scutari as "saving the British Army" and, in so doing, creating a model for all to follow.[5]

One of the most interesting lessons history has to offer is the insight that the taken-for-granted elements of contemporary life are often the result of hard-won victories. When Nightingale first entered public life during the mid-nineteenth century, there were few women on the stage. At that time women were many years away from attaining equal status under the law in any country in the world. In England and the United States religiously inspired activism provided the sole opportunity for women to work among the sick and the poor. In the Protestant world this work was under the careful watch of the pastor with the blessing of the woman's father or husband. Catholic nuns were also busy around the world, building communities and schools and hospitals. Those communities of women still had to negotiate the male terrain of church authorities in the figures of the priests who served as their confessors, and the bishops, who wielded enormous power and demanded their obedience. Thus the very idea of a female profession was in and of itself an entirely radical notion in the mid-nineteenth century, and it was to remain so for the best part of the century that followed. Nightingale's endeavors to build a respectable secular profession for women through the development of training programs for nurses, who would then lead the reform of the hospital, was a breakthrough moment for nursing as it evolved from its previous confines as either religiously motivated or stigmatized as domestic work.

In compiling this book, we have sought to take key elements of the Nightingale story and legacy and bring fresh analyses from leading scholars and thinkers in the field. The aim has been to provide both an update on the scholarship in several areas—the story of Nightingale in the Crimean War, her influence on the colonies of the British Empire, her contribution to statistical sciences, and her impact on the American nursing story—and a review of the current state of play with respect to the endless historiographical myths around her. The contributors represent a wide range of specialized knowledge on the heterogeneous topic of Florence Nightingale. Scholars, of course, have strongly held views and do not necessarily agree with one another. We do not attempt to adjudicate between competing perspectives in the discussion surrounding Nightingale, believing them to be symptomatic of a lively academic field in which scholars continue to debate the interpretation of sources and the significance of events. If Nightingale did not inspire controversy (and its sister, passion), would we still be interested in her a century after her death? Throughout the book there are shades of interpretation and emphasis that vary among contributors. Was Nightingale an opponent of germ theory? Did she create the new model of nursing from which all modern nursing sprang? Read on and make up your own mind! Our hope is that readers develop an awareness of the nuances of historical scholarship and the complexity of the past, as opposed to seeing it as a set of "facts." Facts, as any good historian knows, are not set in stone but matters of interpretation. Nightingale lived a long time. She was also a prolific correspondent and writer, and thus the historical record from her own hand is plentiful. This surfeit of riches creates its own methodological challenges. Individuals change their views over time, they sometimes contradict themselves, they write their different messages to different audiences, and their words may mean something different to a contemporary reader. Nightingale's persona evolved from a young passionate woman to a politically astute social actor to a much revered icon, and her writings reflect this evolution.

The issue of empire forms one of the subthemes of the book, and in Nightingale's lifetime the word "empire" referred to the section of the world that used to be colored red in atlases—the colonies of the British

Empire. The direct thrust of Nightingale's influence occurred in that particular world. However, it was not contained there. In fact, the impact of Nightingale in Japan and Europe and the Americas generated a virtual second empire to rival the first, where the unifying link was Nightingale and she had morphed from a British figure to an eternal representation of feminine goodness and social virtue.

In addition to providing empirical contributions by American, Canadian, and Australian historians, we decided to introduce a series of more reflective elements to allow the reader the chance to think about Nightingale today, what she represents, and the continuing legacy or impact of her work. Chapters 1 and 7 examine the way Nightingale has provided an organizing frame on which nursing's professional aspirations are constantly recast, the way Nightingale's agenda for nursing reform paradoxically still influences the shape of the profession and its priorities in the twenty-first century, and finally the continuity of mission and purpose from the desk of Nightingale which can be traced through the legacy of the school she founded through the donations to the Nightingale Fund that poured in while she was in Scutari and the Crimea. This mix of empirical, theoretical, and reflective essays provides an innovative approach to exploring the ubiquitous figure of Nightingale and her iconographic as well as her historical significance.

As nursing scholars and leaders who are both trained historians and interested in health policy and the politics of the professions, we see Nightingale as a compelling figure in the development of nursing, as well as a shadow figure that plays beneath the surface of nursing's professional identity, public standing, and position within the health care professions. Despite the many profound changes in the delivery of health care over the last hundred years, the transformation in education systems around the world, and the revolution in the workplace in terms of gender politics (at least in Western countries), nursing remains resolutely gendered— with well under 10 percent male participation in the profession overall in the United States, Canada, and Japan and not significantly more in the United Kingdom. The International Council of Nurses, the organization that has represented nursing around the world since 1899, has never had a male president, although for the first time there is now a male executive director. Other elements of the Nightingale vision for nursing remain part of the nursing DNA, not the least of which is the vocational element of nursing work that so many nurses, and perhaps even more members of the public, value about the profession. As the American historian Susan

Reverby observes, nurses are ordered to care in a society that does not value caring.[6] Perhaps much of the fascination with Nightingale is like the public fascination with nursing itself. For despite the great advances in medical science and treatment the patient's full recovery continues to rely on good basic nursing. In fact, Nightingale's one-hundred-fifty-year-old observation still stands: "If a patient is cold, if he has fever, if he is sick after taking food, if he has a bedsore, it is generally not the fault of the disease but of want of good nursing."[7]

How can what was clearly established as a "female" profession break that template to become simply a profession? How too does the ghost of Nightingale shape the professional identities of contemporary nurses for good and bad? In chapter 1 Sioban Nelson examines the power of the idea of Nightingale and the way in which different groups of nurses and other health reformers have over the years attached themselves to her idea or image in order to advance the place of women in society or an agenda for social activism or reform. This chapter uses Benedict Anderson's idea of the "imagined community" to look at the way a Nightingale imperative emerged and was sustained around the world. Nelson argues that under the cloak of Nightingale, whose respectability and noble intentions were without question, it has been possible to advocate for greater professional autonomy for women—an agenda that was controversial in nineteenth-century Britain and remains controversial in many countries of the world today.

In the second chapter the Canadian historian Carol Helmstadter reexamines the landmark event in the creation and immortalization of Florence Nightingale. She re-creates for the reader the complex and competing world of midcentury Victorian Britain and the way in which religion and class shaped and defined the social context of work and politics. The sectarian "intrigues" that bedeviled Nightingale's work during the Crimean War and the influence they had on shaping Nightingale the politician are laid out in fascinating detail.

The third chapter takes the story to the next stage as the Australian historian Judith Godden looks at the empire that Nightingale created from the private space of her bedroom. There, through her tireless correspondence, trained nurses began to have an impact on hospital reform right out to the edges of the British Empire. It was the empire that seeded further empires of trained nurses throughout the colonies and over the course of the following two or three decades reshaped the work of nurses and the face of the modern hospital.

The fourth chapter picks up the story in the United States, where as Joan Lynaugh demonstrates, Nightingale's ideas were taken up in a highly particular way. There a different model of nursing education took root—in the universities—and professionalization and formal education became core values for American nurses.

Chapter 5 changes the tone of the collection with a myth-buster approach to the commonplace errors that abound about Nightingale. The Canadian women's studies scholar Lynn McDonald has taken on the mammoth task of editing Nightingale's full collected works. This set of volumes, sixteen when complete, is a remarkable resource for Nightingale scholars and makes the overwhelming quantity of Nightingale's writings accessible to students and researchers alike. In the course of undertaking this work, McDonald has come across a number of what she argues are consistent errors or misrepresentations about Nightingale.

The next chapter, by Eileen Magnello, examines the mathematical side of Nightingale's brain. In an absorbing account of the relationship between Nightingale and the emergent science of statistics we see the way that Nightingale's interest in data shaped her thinking and provided her with a remarkable ability to see the potential of methodology for politics and policy.

The last word goes to Anne Marie Rafferty and Rosemary Wall. Rafferty, as dean of the Florence Nightingale School of Nursing and Midwifery, sits (literally) at Nightingale's desk—a card table, now used as a writing desk. Rafferty and Wall reflect on the use of Nightingale as an icon for nursing, past and present. They discuss the relevance of Nightingale for the future of nursing, from recruitment to curriculum to professional identity, and for the future of health care generally.

This book aims to reach a wide audience of historians and scholars, graduate nursing students and faculty, and members of the nursing profession. It also sets out to engage the diverse population of Nightingale enthusiasts, people who are inspired by a remarkable woman who led a remarkable life, a woman whose legacy has entered the very fabric of one of the world's biggest and most complex professions. Still enduring the stigma of low-status, feminized domestic work, nurses nonetheless are consistently ranked highly in opinion polls as reliable and worthy of public esteem. The contradictions of high-value low-status work, of complex routine technical work, of virtue versus knowledge bedevil nursing today, no less than a century ago. Reexamining Nightingale is one way to make sense of it all.

THE NIGHTINGALE IMPERATIVE

SIOBAN NELSON

I solemnly pledge myself before God and in the presence of this assembly: To pass my life in purity and to practice my profession faithfully. I will abstain from whatever is deleterious and mischievous, and will not take or knowingly administer any harmful drug. I will do all in my power to elevate the standard of my profession, and will hold in confidence all personal matters committed to my keeping and all family affairs coming to my knowledge in the practice of my profession. With loyalty will I endeavor to aid the physician in his work, and devote myself to the welfare of those committed to my care.

(The Nightingale Pledge)

On 15 August 1945, a short time after the emperor's national radio broadcast announced the unconditional surrender of Japan, a group of nurses at a military hospital in Hiroshima gathered at the order of their commanding officer, the chief medical officer. The young women, exhausted and terrified after nearly two weeks of unimaginable horror, had helplessly witnessed the mass destruction and human suffering following the dropping of the world's first atomic bomb, "Little Boy," at 8:15 a.m. on 6 August. Over those nine days they had seen thousands die (piteously begging for water), they had nursed patients through horrific burn and trauma injuries, and finally, as a mysterious rash began to appear on the bodies of survivors, they had watched as many began to suddenly collapse and die. But the darkest hour came with the emperor's broadcast of surrender. It was an announcement that caused disbelief, panic, and then despair in the city. Such a wave of suicides swept the military hospitals and bases that nurses were forced to hide knives and swords from the men. With the unthinkable capitulation of Japan to its enemies, it seemed that the world was sinking into chaos. All shared the dread of an occupying army and the fear of American soldiers, who were expected to exact a terrible retribution on Japan's citizens. In a preemptive act to restore order to the hospital and dissuade the nurses from running home to their families, the chief medical officer at the Hiroshima Army Red Cross Hospital gathered the nurses and gave them a surprising order: he commanded that they recite the Nightingale Pledge.[1] His tactic worked. According to veteran nurses interviewed by Ryoko O'Hara in her compelling study of nursing at the center of the cataclysm, the pledge seemed to settle the nurses' terror, to remind them of their duty and purpose, and to give them the courage to continue. Under orders, the nurses recited the pledge aloud twice a day for the next week.[2]

How is it that the foreign words, written in 1893 by American nurses in honor of an Englishwoman, could hold such power for Japanese nurses at the very height of nationalist and anti-Western feeling in Japan? What is it about Nightingale and what she represents for nurses around the world that allows the very idea of Nightingale to transcend era and culture to give identity and meaning to professional nursing? Why was the Nightingale story such a fundamental scaffold for the development of nursing around the world, and how did that universal framework function to drive the local nursing agenda, even in situations as exceptional and anti-British as defeated Japan? This chapter is an attempt to answer those questions. In exploring these concerns I am less interested in the elements of the Nightingale story per se and more concerned with the persistent prominence of Nightingale in nursing history and in the identity narratives of nurses around the world. What I am endeavoring to uncover is the role the *idea* of Nightingale has played as a transnational unifying discourse for nurse reformers over time and the way in which the Nightingale narrative continues to be invoked as a legitimizing discourse by nurses across the world to advance the nursing profession and to reform health care.

Over the past one hundred fifty years the Nightingale story has provided discursive energy to power a wide range of nursing stories, offering a consistent reference point for stories that relay the development of national nursing professions or education initiatives, or heroic national stories of war service or nursing during disasters. The secret to the impressive shelf life of the Nightingale ideal, the fact that Nightingale has become synonymous with nursing (of the selfless and dedicated kind), I argue, is a testimony to the malleability of her story to fit multiple audiences and political agendas.

Stories of historical figures are always stories of their times, and enduring figures such as Florence Nightingale have managed to move beyond the locale that produced them to enter the sustaining realm of identity politics, where they remain an integral part of the key stories that are told and retold for successive generations. In her methodological essays in *The Uses and Abuses of History* Margaret MacMillan, Canadian historian and warden of St. Antony's College, Oxford, argues that history plays a major role in the legitimation of ideas, political movements, and nations.[3] Examples abound of the way history can be mustered as a powerful mechanism to silence opposition, justify tyranny, or harness emotion. Common offenders are political leaders. President George W. Bush's supporters found solace through the invocation of parallels with President Harry Truman, who was much maligned by contemporaries but respected by posterity. The Truman analogy was a face-saving salve for the Bush dynasty (despite the fact Truman was a Democrat!).[4] Likewise, Russian leader Josef Stalin's assertion of his destiny to finally fulfill the mandate of the czarist empire, through the expansion of Soviet territory after World War II, provided a patriotic and unifying discursive claim to justify acts of Soviet aggression and self-interest.[5]

MacMillan also points to less profound but no less problematic uses of history. She warns against the dangers of conjuring up an imagined and uncomplicated past full of nostalgic renderings of history that reduce historical actors to easily recognizable good or bad characters, and smooth out the uncomfortable wrinkles of the past by recounting clear injustices with unambiguous remedies. When compared with the complexity and ethical ambiguity of the present, these kinds of histories provide the discursive equivalent of comfort food. For instance, MacMillan sees the recent surge in popularity of movies, novels, and television programs telling World War II stories as symptomatic of contemporary moral ambiguity over the war in Iraq and fears of terrorism. World War II, she argues, was the last good war. Good fought evil, and good prevailed. Today a confused and anxious Western world takes comfort in the noble narrative of World War II, when our parents or grandparents knew what they were doing and why.[6]

For nurses, the uses and abuses of history are just as widespread. There are multiple nursing histories that chronicle a progressivist narrative of reform and development—the "steady progress toward the light" view of history that offers a comforting pat on the back to the visionaries and energetic leaders of the past. Among these are the classic "before and after" images popular in the nineteenth century that compare the drunken, dirty, and dishonest nurse, characterized by Charles Dickens as Sairey Gamp, with the young, bright, and honest "Nightingale" who has transformed nursing and the hospital. There are also tales of dedication and selflessness in wartime and other emergencies when nurses had a major role, perhaps the only women to have done so, in landmark national events such as frontline nurses during World War I or the Vietnam War or as POWs during World War II. But of all the stories one encounters when reading nursing history what stands head and shoulders above the rest is the overriding theme of Florence Nightingale and the movement for the reform of nursing that began with her work in the Crimean War. Whether the topic is education or practice, the profession or hospital reform, the beginning of the new day for nursing, from which all our current days are measured, is the time Nightingale spent in Crimea and Turkey ground-testing her ideas on the scientific management of the sick. This dramatic episode in British history fueled Nightingale's remarkable worldwide reputation as the founder of modern nursing and launched her as one of the great stars of the Victorian era.

The link between the first formal training school for nurses at St. Thomas' Hospital, London, which was established by Nightingale in 1860, and the future development of nursing around the world was a strategic one. Both the idea of formal training for nurses and the ideal of the Nightingale nurse merged over the course of the nineteenth century as the message was spread in three waves. First, there was the phenomenal orb of Nightingale's personal influence. The views of Nightingale, a leading thinker and respected member of the English intelligentsia, were sought on all manner of issues: military nursing and hospital design, the medical education of women, the management of Aboriginal health in Western Australia, and sanitation issues all around the world. She also fielded endless requests for information on nursing and nursing education and hospital management. She advised both Linda Richards, America's first trained nurse, and Elizabeth Blackwell, America's first woman doctor. She gave detailed advice on hospital and sanitary organization during the American Civil War, as well as advised, and was subsequently decorated by, both sides during the Franco-Prussian War.[7] She was a prolific correspondent and provided sound and well-researched advice to all. Her influence in and of itself over the course of her ninety-year life was immense.

Second, we may add to this realm of influence the impact of the Nightingale nurses trained at St. Thomas' who on graduation took with them this particular brand of nursing and hospital management to new hospitals and infirmaries in Britain and throughout the empire (with mixed success; see chapters 3 and 5). Following these St. Thomas' Nightingales came the third wave, late in the nineteenth century, of nurses who were products of the schools established by the first-wave Nightingales, providing a steady stream of English Nightingales to the colonies and beyond.

Thus Nightingale created a movement in the true sense of the term, and the power and legitimacy of these Nightingales stemmed from the authentic connection with the woman herself. By the dawn of the twentieth century, when Nightingale, in her eighties, was still engaged in correspondence, there had been more than thirty years of her personal influence and that of her nurses in all corners of the world. Remarkably, it would have been inconceivable for a conversation on nursing and hospital reform to have occurred anywhere in the world without her views being taken into account one way or another. It is thus no surprise to find that the story of Nightingale turns up in all parts of globe, from the discussions on the organization of nursing in the British colonies to the debates over nursing reform in pre–World War I France, from missionary outposts in Japan to the Catholic countries of Latin America.[8] It is not simply a question of the legacy of Nightingale, what one finds in late nineteenth- and early twentieth-century developments in nursing is a Nightingale imperative. Both the first wave reformers of nursing in the nineteenth century and members of newly established professional communities in the twentieth century were driven by this Nightingale imperative to see themselves as part of a self-conscious movement to establish the profession of nursing worldwide.

The English Nurse: Nightingale in the British Empire

The British social reform movement (1870 to 1930) spearheaded key social and political reforms in the areas of health, education, public policy, and the development of democracy. Although the movement for nursing reform tended for the most part to avoid political association, it encapsulated a number of the core tenets of a progressive agenda: advancing the role of women so that they were able to play a vital part in the development of society, improvement in education, health reform, and progress in civic institutions. Responding to Nightingale's clarion call, under the banner of nursing and service to humanity, women were finally able to take a leading part in reforming a key nineteenth-century social institution—the hospital—and advancing the health of the nation.

As a monumental figure of Victorian England, a reformer and veteran of the Crimean War, Nightingale provided a quintessentially British figure around whom colonizers and colonized could share a common memory and a cause to advance both their societies and the empire as a whole.[9] Across the British Empire the agenda espoused by Nightingale for the reform of nursing was embraced with enthusiasm as colonists were eager to share the glory of one of the empire's leading lights. It was for this reason that the Nightingale Fund for the reform of nursing, set up during the Crimean War (1853–56), was so generously subscribed to by colonists, such as the people of the Colony of New South Wales (Australia), and why Nightingale was continually besieged with requests to send a team of her new nurses to advance the reform of hospitals and nursing. For Nightingale, the generosity of the public toward the Nightingale Fund had created a debt that, in her own words, she would "feign repay" through the export of trained nurses charged with establishing nursing schools throughout the empire.[10]

In the late 1860s, when Nightingale was at the height of her post-Crimean prominence and graduates from St. Thomas' were just beginning to make an impact in the British world, Hilary Bonham Carter created a series of statues in the likeness of Nightingale which were sent to select places around the world. These statues were a small prop in the "Englishization" of nursing that took place in the last three decades of the nineteenth century as part of the nursing reform movement. Over that period, nursing moved from being generally synonymous with menial and degraded labor to a popular and esteemed feminine profession with champions from the highest echelons of society. Nightingale's own prestige and vocational integrity were key elements in this process. Respectable nursing became English nursing, and trappings and icons that symbolically connected nursing to Nightingale proliferated. Enthusiasm for nursing reform not only brought progressive British developments to

the periphery of the empire (and throughout the world) but also signi-
fied an affirmation of British values.

The Sydney Infirmary in New South Wales, Australia, began as a convict institution—that is, convict inmates served as nurses for the original penal settlement of Sydney. In 1868, when the Nightingale nurses
arrived, the Infirmary still carried the stigma of its convict heritage and
was staffed by poorly educated servant nurses. Following a direct request from the colonial secretary, Sir Henry Parkes, for a team of Nightingale nurses to lead the reform of Australian nursing, and mindful of the
colonial support for the Nightingale Fund for the development of nursing training, Nightingale sent a team of nurses, who arrived in late 1868
under the leadership of Lucy Osburn.[11] The English nurses found the
Irish servant nurses slovenly and ignorant by English standards. They
were deeply shocked at the unkempt appearance of the nurses, and thus
lessons in personal grooming, hairdressing tips, and the purchase of hand
mirrors were priorities on the long list of reforms required of Sydney's
local nursing workforce.[12] If the English nurses thought the Irish Australian staff needed a serious makeover, it appears that the Irish Australian
nurses for their part thought they were being taken over by a strange
religious movement headed by Nightingale.[13] According to Osburn, the
nurses were greatly impressed by the arrival of the three Bonham Carter
statuettes of Nightingale. With her hands poised to give a blessing and
eyes raised to heaven, Nightingale had fully entered the realm of the su-
pernatural. For these old-style nurses, finding the statues in prominent
positions overlooking the wards and the nurses' daily work was further
evidence of Nightingale's canonization.[14]

The early beatification of Nightingale in the eyes of the Irish nurses
at the Sydney Infirmary was only one part of the symbolic constitution
of empire enacted by the diasporic community. Monuments to Queen
Victoria and imperial heroes such as Admiral Horatio Nelson, victor
of the Battle of Trafalgar in 1805, dotted the world from Montreal to
Cape Town, as key elements in the making and remaking of the British
world. Even a century later the phenomenon continued through movements such as the "transnational outrage" and proliferation of monuments and namings in honor of English nurse Edith Cavell,[15] executed
by the Germans during World War I in 1915. Cavell was executed by the
Germans for espionage, namely, for helping British soldiers make their
way home from inside occupied Belgium. The sensation surrounding
her death proved a remarkable tool for recruitment propaganda during

World War I. It was sustained by nationalist and British fervor between the wars and then reenergized by anti-German sentiment with World War II.[16] As Katie Pickles argues, anger and grief at the death of Cavell functioned to both express and constitute Britishness:

> The common sentiment expressed at Cavell's death met with common initiatives by groups of elite women who held a shared sense of being branches of Britishness. Outside of Britain, largely urban elites, well connected Anglo-Celtic women from wealthy families, in particular in the imperial cities of Toronto, Melbourne, Sydney and Brisbane, set about copying the example set by the British and Continental commemoration of Cavell. These female imperialists claimed Cavell as the model British citizen, and an appropriate role model for fostering Britishness in their respective dominions.[17]

The story of Edith Cavell is particularly illustrative of the way remembrance is fueled by contemporary needs. Hers was one of the most recognizable names throughout the British world and in France, Italy, and Belgium for decades, yet she is scarcely known today, the story retaining few echoes for contemporary sensibilities.

In many parts of the world it was the Britishness of Nightingale that allowed her to remain a powerful figure in times of war or instability. But unlike Lord Nelson or Edith Cavell, Nightingale was a symbol for all seasons: she could be a saintly figure for a feminine vocation, a determined reformer for an agenda of change, or a national icon for patriotic service.

Either directly or by association, Nightingale provided the legitimacy for a reform agenda for nursing. Her name was synonymous with respectability and reform of the most English type. When Queen Victoria's son Prince Alfred was injured in an assassination attempt by a supposed Fenian in Sydney in 1868, weeks after the first group of Nightingale nurses had arrived in the colony to begin the reform of nursing, the newspapers gushed relief that although the incident was a terrible shame on the colony, thankfully Sydney could boast an English Nightingale, one of "our fair Sisters of Charity," to care for him during his recovery.[18]

By the turn of the century a new English nurse, the colonial service nurse, took up the mantle of Nightingale in the parts of the empire where Europeans were few. These nurses were part of the extensive network of British civil servants who worked across the empire, which in 1900 represented a vast portion of territory from Canada to India, the African colonies, Australia and New Zealand, and the Malay Peninsula—a third of the world. In Singapore, as described in the official history published by the Singaporean government in 2000, the first colonial service nurse freed Singapore from what was portrayed as the worthy but untrained care of the French nuns and introduced modern professional nursing to the colony.[19] Similar stories are played out across the empire, where colonial service nurses, as standard bearers of English nursing practice, aimed to lead colonized peoples to develop British standards of excellence and at the same time make the colonies safe for the colonizers—the British and their families. Historians of gender and colonization such as Ann McGrath and Ann Laura Stoler have examined the common strategies used by colonizers to encourage the settlement of white women in colonial outposts.[20] White women provided a remedy to the danger of racial intermarriage, considered a threat to the civilizing drive of Western colonization, and English nurses, with their high moral standards, training, and respectability, not only created the "civilized" conditions that would support the development of a British way of life but provided the womanpower to do so. Nurses, from the very first group of Nightingales to be sent from England in 1868 to the veritable army of colonial service nurses fifty years later, were certainly viewed as good marriage prospects. In the former case, in Sydney, Lucy Osburn wryly observed the way her English nurses enthusiastically and successfully pursued Australian husbands.[21] In the latter, the marriage of colonial nurses to fellow British subjects in the empire was in fact a measure of success for the service, which actively recruited nurses to the organization by the none-too-subtle lure of potential husbands.[22]

Thus for British subjects in the nineteenth and early twentieth centuries, the power of the Nightingale reform movement was energized by the invocation of Englishness that the reform of nursing entailed. Whether it was the initial patriotic impetus of the Nightingale Fund during the Crimean War or support of progressive and innovative approaches to hospitals and health under the direction of Nightingale-style nurses, an "imagined community" of empire was both created and sustained by participation, however tenuous, in the Nightingale story.

Beyond the Empire

As historian Benedict Anderson so famously declared when talking about nations, "communities are to be distinguished by the style in which they are imagined."[23] Beyond the borders of the British Empire a second imagined community had emerged by the end of the nineteenth century—a nursing community. The establishment of the International Council of Nurses in 1899, under the transatlantic leadership of American feminist Lavinia Dock and Englishwoman Ethel Bedford Fenwick, launched nursing as a profession with a noble destiny: to harness the intellectual and moral energy of women to transform the health and welfare of the world.[24] Female suffrage, the regulation of nursing, and the pursuit of health and human dignity were the cornerstones of this movement. Despite the fact that Nightingale and Bedford Fenwick had not seen eye to eye on a number of issues (most particularly Bedford Fenwick's dearest cause—nursing registration), twenty years after the death of Nightingale the politically astute Bedford Fenwick found the occasion of the demolition of Nightingale's house on South Street the perfect opportunity to invoke Nightingale's name in support of her contemporary cause in a manner that Lucien Lefebre calls "the deification of the present with the aid of the past."[25]

On July 4, 1932, with full pomp and ceremony, students attending the International Course at Bedford College, London, were each presented with a parcel wrapped in national colors (see Figure 1). Each parcel contained a brick from the recently demolished residence at South Street where Nightingale lived from 1865 to 1910. With great pomp and circumstance Bedford Fenwick, president of the International Council of Nurses of Great Britain, declared that these bricks, which hailed from the very room in which Miss Nightingale had spent most of her time, were a gift to the students' homelands. She added, "In owning a Brick from the walls of this sometime sacred room, I feel sure your National Association of Nurses will realize it possesses a treasure far above rubies." The *British Journal of Nursing* reported that the delegates "expressed their sincere pride and pleasure" in possessing the bricks, "from which it was felt nothing was too wonderful to upspring."[26]

Notwithstanding the hubris characteristic of speeches of the time (especially Bedford Fenwick's), the story of the sacred Nightingale bricks is instructive. Reminiscent of the saintly statuettes some sixty years before, the bricks functioned as modern-day relics, providing a Nightingale blessing on the endeavors of the recipient. Proclaimed "a link between the nurses of the world"[27] (albeit with little enthusiasm from "home country nurses"[28]), the bricks were also reserved as gifts to the nurse training schools of hospitals throughout the world. A few made their way to the United States: a Miss A. E. MacDonald, president

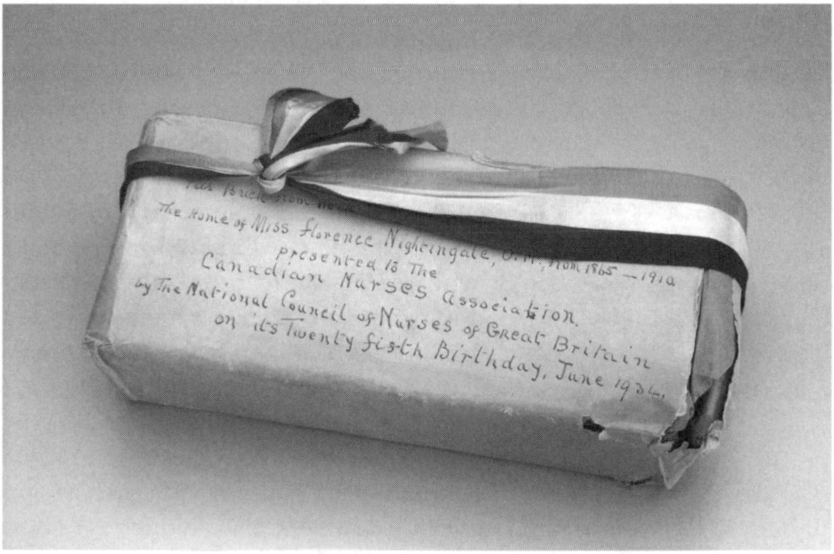

Fig. 1. Commemorative brick from Florence Nightingale's house in South Street Westminster, London. Photo © Canadian Museum of Civilization, 2000.111.425, IMG2009-0326-0005-Dm.

of the Nurses Association for the Gordon Hospital, Plymouth, Massachusetts, received one in 1937.[29] Another is currently held by the Yale University School of Nursing Archive.[30] Mary Breckinridge placed one in the stone chimney of the Margaret Voorhies Haggin Quarters for Nurses at the Hyden Hospital in Kentucky.[31] The overwhelming majority were sent on request to Dominion countries: Canada, Australia, New Zealand, South Africa, and Barbados. Like Breckinridge's brick, they became centerpieces in fireplaces in nurses' homes and hospitals (Royal Melbourne Hospital) or foundation stones of new nurses' homes (Invercargill, New Zealand; Vancouver, Canada) or were sold to raise funds for the Florence Nightingale International Foundation.

The case of the Nightingale house bricks is only a minor tale in the vast repertoire of Nightingale stories, but it is a telling one. The story highlights the importance of a concrete connection with Nightingale and the reflected glory it bestows. For nursing schools as diverse as the Yale School of Nursing, at one of America's premier private universities, and the Royal Melbourne Hospital's Training School, a hospital-based program in Victoria, Australia, to place value on the symbolic identification with Nightingale and what she represents for nursing is testimony not only to the universality of the discourse but also to its malleability. For the traditional-mold Royal Melbourne Hospital, there was pride in being a Nightingale-model nursing training school; for Yale, the appeal did not imply a Nightingale model or even tradition, but leadership, intelligence, and innovation.

As historians Eric Hobsbawm and Terence Ranger argue, traditions are invented in "response to novel situations which take the form of reference to old situations, or which establish their own past by quasi-obligatory repetition."[32] So for nursing organizations such as schools and hospitals, objects from iconic figures such as Nightingale (and there are none more iconic) allow for the establishment of new pasts in which the history of the organization can be seen as part of a natural and highly prestigious tradition. For the organizations involved, evidence of the Nightingale pedigree flows from the imprimatur of objects such as portraits of Nightingale, framed fragments of letters (also ubiquitous), or the South Street bricks.

Lest such overt affection for the memory of Nightingale appear to be an artifact of twentieth-century sentimentalism, there is ample contemporary evidence of continued attachment to practices that affirm a genealogy of nursing education where all paths lead back to Nightingale. Thus in many countries one finds a connection with the Nightingale movement that provides legitimacy and a shared history for nursing around the world.

Community is both created and sustained by shared practices, the invention of traditions, and the inculcation of consistent values. The symbolic recognition that nursing students on graduation are entering into what Patricia Benner would call a practice community, in the Aristotelian sense,[33] has long been achieved through ritual (ceremonial events such as awards, namings, pinnings, cappings, and pledges), through discourse (such as curricula), and through peer-to-peer practices that reinforce group identity and establish the roles of novices and mentors in the cultural system.

There are many ways that these practices can be understood theoretically. Anthropologists can show their importance in the creation of group identity, Pierre Bourdieu's ideas on habitus can be helpfully applied to understand the way a field or domain generates practices that sustain the field,[34] Michel Foucault's work on subjectivity opens the way to think about these practices as possessing their own history and about how their migration from the military domain or the world of the convent brings with it particular subjective elements that in turn shape the personas they then constitute.[35] But however deep one wishes to enter the theoretical territory of ritual and identity formation in nursing, these practices indubitably hold a powerful place in shaping the professional identity of the nurse, and, so often, lead the nurse back to Nightingale.

One compelling ubiquitous example of a shared practice that generates the imagined community of nursing is the Nightingale Pledge. A tradition invented in 1893 in Michigan,[36] it became popular as part of graduation and pinning ceremonies in the United States over the course of the twentieth century as a parallel to the Hippocratic Oath taken by medical graduates.

Throughout the world, particularly in areas influenced primarily by American nursing, the pledge became a core ceremony in the event that symbolized the new nurse's assumption of full professional responsibilities at the completion of her training. As we saw at the beginning of the chapter, even at the center of the Japanese military machine during World War II, Japanese nurses found meaning and purpose in that pledge. Today nurses around the world continue to recite it and across the United States, in the Philippines, in China, India, or Lebanon, young nurses add shaky videos and blurred photos of their pledge ceremony to their MySpace or Facebook pages, rejoicing in the rite of passage it represents.

Part of the power of the Nightingale Pledge is the conscious assertion by novice nurses that they are continuing a tradition, a tradition that involves upholding a system of values and civic mission to serve humanity. The pledge, along with other Nightingale gestures, asserts the primary importance of the noblesse oblige of nursing, and invokes Nightingale's monumental stature as a way of lifting nursing into the realm of higher service and distancing itself from the routine service work with which it remains stigmatized. The issue of the legitimacy of nursing as a profession, despite apparent advances in North America and Europe in recent decades, remains key to both the self-image and the public image of nursing. Even in countries where women have achieved legal parity with men, nursing continues to suffer from the stigma of lowly women's work. In fact, in late 2009 the announcement that English nursing was moving to degree-entry to practice generated a public debate in leading newspapers about the professional status of nursing and questioned the need for higher levels of education.[37] In countries where the status of women remains low, efforts to legitimate the nursing profession continue to be closely linked with the struggle for women's rights. For the nursing profession to flourish, women need educational opportunities, a career path within the health-care system, and a voice in health policy and service development. The legitimation of the nursing profession involves the evergreen tenets of the nineteenth-century progressive agenda: advancing the role of women so that they may play a vital role in the development of society, improvement in education, health reform, and progress in civic institutions.

Invoking the Nightingale tradition foregrounds the fact that nursing is a form of higher service to humanity. It is respectable and embraces the highest ideals of a profession, as opposed to representing a technical supportive role that is subordinate to medicine. Around the world the Nightingale name provides a kind of talismanic ability to address the same issues that confronted the nineteenth-century nurses in their efforts to create nursing as a respectable and scientific profession for women. Nineteenth-century nurses needed to overcome the stigma of working with bodies (particularly male bodies) as well as the stigma of working with the sick, work that was once the province of the lowest of servants. They also had to overcome the widely held view that women needed to be supervised and under male control at all times and that respectability could not be maintained in a workplace that included men and women. Today these issues remain powerful obstacles to nursing in many parts of the world. In countries where women have not attained equal status under the law, the idea of a self-regulating profession where women form the majority is radical in and of itself. Even in parts of the world where the numbers of male nurses are higher than in the United States or Britain, the gendered history of the profession continues to characterize it as feminized and subordinate.

Strengthening nursing to strengthen the health-care system is a contemporary plank of the International Council of Nurses and associated national nursing organizations,[38] and in countries in Africa, Asia, and the Middle East the invocation of the near saintly Nightingale provides an acceptable and legitimizing tone for a potentially radical antipatriarchal discourse. Strengthening nursing involves the development of nursing as a self-regulated independent profession, that is, a profession that is not directly under medical or government jurisdiction. It involves support for nursing education that is conducted by nurses, not by physicians, and a regulatory framework for the profession that is governed by nurses. None of these elements is particularly derived from Nightingale, save the overall premise that a good health-care system (not that she would have used that term) relies on good scientific principles and well-trained nurses. Nonetheless, there is a discursive power in combining the Nightingale tradition, which invokes higher service to humanity, respectability, and the highest ideals of a profession, with a contemporary professionalizing agenda.

Studies of history and memory tell us less about historical detail than they do about collective memory and the place of key events in identity narratives. Oral historians know too well that memory can deceive, and there are many examples of memory not fitting the historical record.[39] For instance, an oral history project that compared the data from interviews taken of Londoners during the London Blitz of World War II with interviews taken decades later found that individuals genuinely recall the war as a time when there was sharing and camaraderie against a common enemy—notions that were entirely absent from the wartime interview data. What this disconnect between stories over time tells us is that historical memory is collective, shaped by narratives that make us who we are. Stories of oppression become the tales of our wounds, stories of triumph become our victories. Stories that stand the test of time continue to serve a function. Nationalist stories do not only maintain identity but create it, or as Ernest Gellner argues, "nationalism is not the awakening of nation to self consciousness, it invents nations where they do not exist."[40]

In the British world the use of school curriculum to promote ruling discourses of Britishness and to encourage good citizenship in the next generation has been appropriately termed the "imperial curriculum."[41] The function of history in this curriculum is to celebrate imperial achievements and to erase local or resistance narratives. As Ashcroft argues, "This capacity to interpellate imperial subjects, to inculcate a particular view of the world, a particular morality, a range of aesthetic, ethical, political, and social values in the colonized is a very good demonstration of hegemony."[42] In much the same way as the imperial curriculum functioned to induct citizens of the empire, the transmission of values and an agreed-on history furnish elements of professional formation in professions such as law or medicine or nursing. In the core history curricula once taught as a standard part of hospital-based nursing programs around the world, there was a central place for Nightingale, the Crimean War, and the reform of nursing from the dark to the modern age through her work and life. Although hospital-based training programs have been replaced by modern academic curricula, in which the focus tends to be on ethics and contemporary values, core content concerning Nightingale is still a frequent part of nursing curricula around the world. In a review of nursing curricula in Australia, Brazil, the United States, and Canada, it was found that the essential elements were a strong emphasis on the nineteenth-century reform movement and the establishment of nursing education in each country.[43] Thus the history of nursing as it forms part of nursing curricula tends to reproduce a familiar heroic narrative that anchors the reform and progressive development of nursing with the movement initiated by Nightingale in the nineteenth century. Today, no less so than in the hospital-based programs of the early and mid-twentieth century, recurrent tropes of service, respectability, and leadership continue to anchor the professional formation of nurses as part of a Nightingale tradition.[44]

A New World Order? Nightingale in the Twenty-first Century

When we are dealing with a figure of such emblematic importance as Florence Nightingale, it is important to give space for multiple meanings and interpretations. It is clear that the pedestal on which Nightingale stands has been subject to some shaky moments over the past one hundred fifty years. At times, such as during the world wars and in the minds of pro-British members of the failing empire, Nightingale's standing among the British elite has been symbolically important and her name has invoked a set of values associated with membership in the empire—leadership, whiteness, Britishness. For others and for other times, it is Nightingale the reformer who stirs the identification. Her tireless campaigns to improve sanitation, fight disease, and decrease mortality among the poor, particularly her commitment to sanitary reform in India, allow for her name to be invoked for an entirely different cause—the cause of science, of reform, of progress. For nurses, the name of Nightingale has been avowed and rejected in turn by competing forces. In recent years in the United Kingdom, union leaders have called for a new symbol for nursing.[45] Looking for someone who resonates with contemporary values and finding Nightingale lacking, revisionist critics of the official story spawned a new set of myths about the character of Nightingale's mysterious disease (was it syphilis?), her relationships (was she mentally unstable? was there a deep scandal?), and her contribution to nursing (was she even the architect of modern nursing at all?).

Despite the misgivings, the correctives, and the overcorrections of the traditional Nightingale story, the Lady with a Lamp does not appear to be any further from center stage than she has ever been. New biographies are still coming out each year, her birthday is celebrated around the world by nursing groups and health-care providers as part of Nurses' Week, and her name alone retains the power to evoke a higher cause for nursing work. A recent example of the power of Nightingale as a signifier of all that is noble and good in nursing comes from Barbara Dossey and colleagues with the establishment of the Nightingale Initiative for Global Health (NIGH).[46] They characterize Nightingale as "a pro-active, vocal conscience for the health of humanity." Holding closely to the template established over the course of the past century, the NIGH initiative has even developed its own version of the Nightingale Pledge, rescripting it as a prayer for a better world:

Our Nightingale Prayer
Today, our world needs healing and to be rekindled with Love.
Once, Florence Nightingale lit her beacon of lamplight to comfort the
    wounded
and her Light has blazed a path of service across a Century to us,
through her example and through the countless Nurses and Healers
who have followed in her footsteps.
Today, we celebrate the flame of Florence Nightingale's Legacy.
Let that same Light be rekindled to burn brightly in our hearts.
Let us take up our own Lanterns of Caring, each in our own ways.
To more brightly walk our own paths of service to the World.
To more clearly share our own Noble Purpose with each other.
May Human Caring become the Lantern for the 21st Century.
May we better learn to care for ourselves,
for each other and for all Creation.
Through our Caring, may we be the Keepers of that Flame.
That Our Spirits may burn brightly
to kindle the hearts of our children and great-grandchildren
as they too follow in these footsteps.[47]

The mission of NIGH is to inform and empower nurses and other health-care workers and educators to become "21st Century Nightingales," working in the local, national, and global community to build a healthy world. Part of its mandate is "encouraging individual initiative and cooperative action toward these ends by highlighting the life of Florence Nightingale and the lives of other nurses and health care workers—past and present—who have devoted themselves to building a healthy world."[48]

In this version of Nightingale we find an agent of change and a committed activist (to use contemporary terms). The organizers, like Bedford Fenwick with her Nightingale bricks eighty years earlier, have seen the utility of mustering the past for a future goal.

The reform of nursing and the Nightingale movement emerged from fertile ground. Over the decades following the Crimean War, hospital reform became increasingly necessary as modern medicine evolved and its demands outstripped the skills and competencies of old-style semiliterate nurses. Although this development set the scene for power struggles between medicine and nursing as to who was going to manage the modern hospital—the Nightingale-style matron or the medical superintendent—it also meant that progressive physicians were some of the strongest advocates of trained nursing and improvements to nurses' working conditions. In fact, from Melbourne to Tokyo to the London teaching hospitals, it was typically physicians who realized that modern medical care was being held back by the lack of trained nurses.[49] Nightingale provided a solution to this conundrum. A woman of class and means dedicated herself not only to the care of the sick but also to ensuring that nursing care would itself be revolutionized by respectable women who could lead nursing toward a new era of professionalization and dignity. The nineteenth-century barriers that needed to be overcome included the stigma attached to the work as unclean and immoral due to its association with low domestic work, the opposition of families to their daughters' independent pursuit of a calling (or career), and the need to organize training schools to ensure that nurses brought the requisite knowledge to the direct care and the organization of care of the sick.

The gendered divide between nursing and medicine, which placed nursing as supportive and dependent, has in turn continued to play out in the politics of twenty-first-century health care. At the same time, the social stigma against nursing as glorified servant's work has proven an even tougher obstacle to nursing's professional development than conflict with physicians or challenges with regulation and education. It could be argued that the persistence of nursing's obsession with Nightingale lies with the lack of resolution of these gendered tensions over virtue versus knowledge or education versus what Nightingale called "character." But whatever glass ceiling in professional status this vocational aspect of the profession still creates in North America, Australia, or Europe, in parts of the world where the position of women remains subject to the same patriarchal restrictions as those experienced by Victorian women, the Nightingale story continues to act as a talisman for respectability and feminine power. In the name of Nightingale, women can pursue professional autonomy, and care of the sick can be lifted from the technical or domestic realm to play a critical role in the health-care system. Today, no less than in the nineteenth century, under the watchful eye of Miss Nightingale the care of male bodies by young women can be pure and noncorrupting and women's professional aspirations can serve the goals of civic duty and patriotism.[50] A century after the death of Nightingale the ties that bind her name to nursing remain as strong as ever.

NAVIGATING THE POLITICAL STRAITS IN THE CRIMEAN WAR

CAROL HELMSTADTER*

Florence Nightingale was well steeped in politics when she and her team of nurses set out for the East in 1854.[1] She hailed from a political family. Her grandfather, William Smith, member of Parliament (MP) from 1784 to 1830, was a leader of the radical party that led the movements to reform Parliament, abolish the slave trade, and pass the Catholic Emancipation Act. Smith himself was the key architect of the repeal of the Test and Corporations acts. These reforms were all landmarks in the history of early nineteenth-century England. Nightingale was fifteen when her grandfather died and knew him well because he was devoted to his grandchildren and visited them regularly. Nightingale's father, W. E. Nightingale, served as a county administrator. In 1832 he and her uncle, John Bonham Carter, also an MP, were major organizers of Lord Palmerston's campaign for reelection. Palmerston, a family friend and next-door neighbor, had been foreign secretary and would later become one of the significant nineteenth-century prime ministers. In 1834 W. E. Nightingale stood for Parliament himself but was not elected.[2]

As Barbara Dossey observes, Nightingale had an understanding of politics that children of successful political families often develop: "an

* I thank Associated Medical Services Toronto, Canada, for generously funding much of the research on which this chapter is based, and Lynn McDonald, editor of *The Collected Works of Florence Nightingale,* for access to its electronic archives.

early knowledge of local and national political processes, the psychology of politics, where the levers of power are and how to win."[3] On a nongovernmental level, as superintendent of the Hospital for Gentlewomen in Harley Street in 1853–54, Nightingale worked closely and well with medical men and learned how to deal with a committee of ladies, some of whom she considered petty and incompetent.[4] The Crimean War, however, catapulted Nightingale onto the international scene and made her a government-appointed officer who had to deal personally with the War Office. As a woman with no political rights, Nightingale had a knowledge of politics that stemmed from supporting election campaigns, meeting socially with top government ministers, and studying their policy. Her position as a government official, involved in implementing government policy and making decisions that affected it, would demand a somewhat different approach.

The Political Nature of Nightingale's Mission

The occasion for Nightingale's government commission was the fierce public outcry over the lack of care for the wounded and dying during the Crimean War. Following the battle of the Alma on 20 September 1854, the press, now able to receive communiqués by telegraph, printed graphic details of the sufferings of the soldiers. The British army's medical department compared very unfavorably with that of the French. The Sisters of Charity, who provided the nursing in the French base hospitals, were especially admired, and the English government came under intense pressure to improve the army's nursing care. Sidney Herbert, who was in the War Office and a personal friend of Florence Nightingale, approached her to organize a team of female nurses to work in the base hospitals in Turkey.[5]

Nightingale's assignment was humanitarian, but its primary impetus was therefore very political—to quell the outrage over the government's conduct of the war. Her orders reflected this: the War Office instructed her, first, to insist that her nurses implicitly obey the orders of the doctors and purveyors and, second, to prevent all religious disputes.[6] The politicians were concerned with obedience to the doctors and purveyors because neither the military doctors nor the purveyors had requested nurses. The Duke of Newcastle, the minister of war, later explained that the War Office had considered employing female nurses before the army left the country, but the military men were "very adverse" to the idea because when ordinary hospital nurses had been tried in the past, the women were "addicted to drink" and, Newcastle said, were "often more callous to the sufferings of the soldiers than those male attendants who had been employed more recently." However, when Nightingale agreed to organize the venture, the government decided to forge ahead. Nevertheless, the ministry was afraid the military doctors would not accept Nightingale and her team when they arrived in Scutari.[7]

It is easy to see why the War Office was concerned about collaboration with the army doctors, but why was Nightingale's second instruction, to prevent religious discord, so important? This order reflected the centrality of religion and the intensely political nature of sectarian controversy in mid-nineteenth-century English life. There was a long tradition of anti-Catholicism in England, dating from the Reformation, when Henry VIII rejected the primacy of the pope and made himself head of the Church of England. The Glorious Revolution of 1688 dethroned a Roman Catholic king. The Act of Settlement of 1701 disinherited more than fifty legitimate heirs to the throne in order to crown the Protestant (and very German) George I. What was called the "Protestant Constitution" allowed toleration and practice of differing religious opinions, but the seventeenth-century Test and Corporations acts prohibited non-Anglicans from exercising political power: only Anglicans could hold national and local public office.[8] Religious freedom did not bring political equality with it, which explains why sectarian issues were so contentious in Parliament.

In the campaign to break the Anglican monopoly of political power, William Smith was the Dissenters' most influential political spokesman.[9] The repeal of the Test and Corporations acts in 1828 and Catholic Emancipation in 1829 allowed Dissenters and Roman Catholics to officially hold public office. However, other disabilities remained, and more importantly, intense religious bigotry, on the part of both Roman Catholics and Protestants, continued with greater intensity than ever.[10] Nightingale was keenly sensitive to these sectarian prejudices. In line with her grandfather's radical political position, as superintendent at Harley Street she insisted, against considerable opposition, on admitting patients of all religious faiths and allowing their priests, ministers, and rabbis to visit them.[11]

The union of Ireland and Great Britain in 1800 added another element to national politics, for it put one hundred (and after 1832 one hundred five) new Irish members into Parliament.[12] Both the Aberdeen coalition government, which sent Nightingale to the East and which fell in January 1855, and Palmerston's Whig government, which succeeded it, were dependent on Irish votes, which were integrally tied to the Roman Catholic question. It was therefore a political imperative that Nightingale show no bias toward any religious denomination. The War Department accurately judged Nightingale's two major obstacles: religious disputes and resistance from the doctors. She would come into conflict with the Irish Roman Catholic issue when the militant Mother Francis Bridgeman arrived in Constantinople, and Sir John Hall, unfortunately for Nightingale the army's chief medical officer, would strongly resist Nightingale's presence in the Crimea. The problem was made much more severe when Hall allied himself with Bridgeman.

The Nursing Team

The Political, Religious, and Social Framework of Nightingale's Mission

Nightingale was acutely aware of the resistance she and her nurses might meet. In nineteenth-century England, upper-class women, always called "ladies" to distinguish them from working-class women, were confined to the domestic sphere. Frank Prochaska described this sphere as "the nursery and the sick chamber, the home and the neighborhood, the church and the foot of the cross." The army, quintessentially a man's world, and its hospitals were clearly part of the public sphere. Nursing was a specific attribute of ladies but was appropriately exercised only in the private domain—in the sick chamber, not in public hospitals.[13]

When Herbert asked her to take a team of nurses to the East, Nightingale was already planning to go, "quietly and privately," with three or four nurses. She thought if she took more women the doctors would oppose her.[14] In fact, she went to Scutari not quietly and privately but with great fanfare as the head of thirty-eight government-paid nurses. Although she was thirty-three years old and had total responsibility for a small hospital, Nightingale, like all unmarried ladies, needed her parents' permission to undertake any enterprise. She therefore sent her uncle to her parents' home to get their consent.[15] She also needed a chaperone, another illustration of the severe restrictions Victorian society placed on unmarried daughters. Her old and close friends Charles and Selina Bracebridge agreed to accompany her.[16]

To prevent showing favoritism to any one sect, Nightingale selected nurses from almost every religious denomination in Britain. Compounding her difficulties with conflicting and warring religious loyalties, the nurses came from almost every level of society.[17] The majority were working-class because she specifically asked for experienced hospital nurses, who of course were all working-class women, but there were also middle-class ladies and even two minor aristocrats on her team. The nurses for whom we have reasonable records fall into four groups: approximately 128 working-class women, 9 Anglican sisters, 28 Roman Catholic nuns, and 52 secular ladies.[18]

The multiclass aspect presented a major problem because Victorian society, with what amounted to almost a caste system, segregated ladies from working-class women. Most of the Roman Catholic nuns and all the Anglican sisters were ladies. For Mother Mary Clare Moore, the superior of the Convent of Mercy in Bermondsey, it was very difficult to have her sisters associated with Protestants and working-class nurses. It would be an exercise in mortification, her bishop, Bishop Thomas Grant of Southwark, wrote Moore after she left London. "The very fact of being associated with the [hospital] nurses," she would later write, "who, although respectful to the sisters, were persons of doubtful character and almost daily intoxicated, caused great pain and uneasiness." Conversely, some Protestant women, prime among whom was Nightingale's trusted matron Mrs. Clark, treated the Roman Catholic nuns appallingly.[19]

Herbert told Nightingale that many ladies had offered their services but he thought she was the only lady in England who was capable of meeting the challenges of such a daunting enterprise. He knew the task of ruling the nurses "and introducing system among them" would be very difficult and the work of directing and organizing them enormous. Working collaboratively with the military and medical authorities was yet another problem. But "your own personal qualities," Herbert wrote, "your knowledge and your power of administration, and among greater things your rank and position in society give you advantages in such a work which no other person possesses."[20]

Herbert's weighting of Nightingale's qualifications, placing her social rank above her competencies and nursing experience, was characteristic of the deferential society of the 1850s. And indeed, Herbert had a fair point, for had Eliza Roberts, a working-class nurse whose professional qualifications and expertise far exceeded those of Nightingale,[21] been put in charge of the expedition, it would surely have failed. "She was a splendid nurse and an excellent woman," Nightingale wrote later, "but had no command." Roberts's working-class background, her terrible temper and manners, and her weak literacy skills would have made it impossible for her to cope.[22]

Nightingale met with Herbert on 16 October to discuss the plans, and on 19 October she received her official appointment as Superintendent of the Female Nursing Establishment in the Military Hospitals in Turkey. The government would pay all the costs of the expedition, and Nightingale would have complete control of the nurses, subject to the sanction and approval of the chief medical officer. However, Nightingale alone would select the nurses, determine their assignments, set their various rates of pay, and, if necessary, fire them. She was to keep the number of Roman Catholics in any single hospital at a ratio of one to three.[23]

Recruiting the Nurses

Nightingale now had to find the nurses. She went first to women's organizations. She recruited eight sisters from two of the new Anglican sisterhoods, the Park Village sisters and the Devonport Sisters of Mercy, and six working-class nurses trained by a third Anglican sisterhood, the Order of St. John the Evangelist, or St. John's House, as it was more popularly known. This sisterhood was designed as a training school for nurses and consisted of ladies who were lay sisters and paid, working-class nurses. Many writers have wrongly assumed that the six St. John's House nurses were sisters, but actually they were paid, working-class nurses. In her effort to be nonsectarian, Nightingale also approached Mrs. Fry's Devonshire Square Sisters, a Protestant institution founded by a Quaker, but its board, at this point, was not willing to give Nightingale full control of their nurses. They later sent six nurses to the East. In March 1855, when fifteen nurses were laid low with fever, Nightingale requested more nurses. To make her team more interdenominational, she asked that four to six be Presbyterians.[24]

Bishop Grant immediately saw a political opportunity in Nightingale's expedition: he thought it could give Roman Catholic nuns a chance to demonstrate publicly "how earnest and charitable nuns are and how much they excel all other nurses." In this era of violent denominational warfare, when nuns were harshly discriminated against, Grant thought the sisters' zeal and charity would disarm prejudice. Mother Mary Clare Moore found it "a comfort to know that the Protestant government has consented to employ poor nuns as nurses." Together with Dr. (later Cardinal) Henry Manning, Grant recruited ten nuns, five from Moore's convent and five who ran an orphanage in Norwood. Finally, Nightingale's two friends, Mary Stanley and Elizabeth Herbert, advertised for hospital nurses and hired fourteen. In Paris, en route to Scutari, Nightingale tried unsuccessfully to recruit French nursing sisters from the Order of St. Vincent de Paul.[25]

Like Herbert and Newcastle, Nightingale was concerned by the working-class nurses' lack of discipline and was therefore anxious to keep the party small, especially "in so new a position as a military hospital."[26] In fact, her job would be more complex than organizing the nursing service in one hospital. The Crimean War nurses worked in eleven different hospitals,[27] and further complicating matters, the hospitals opened and closed at various times. And for political reasons, Herbert insisted on forty nurses when Nightingale thought twenty would be more efficient. She somewhat unwillingly agreed to the larger number because she appreciated Herbert's point that more nurses would give the government better publicity.[28]

Nightingale's qualifications as a nurse are well known. Less well known is that while many of the ladies found the strange customs, dirt, rats, and fleas a terrible trial, Nightingale was a seasoned traveler in what the Victorians called the "East" (Egypt) and was well prepared for the horrific living conditions in Scutari. Having traveled in the company of all types of women, she found the heterogeneous nature of her nursing party less of a shock than did many of the more sheltered ladies, for whom living at such close quarters with ladies of different religious denominations as well as the uneducated working-class nurses was a dreadful ordeal. Nightingale's varied experiences included, among others, sitting in an Egyptian harem drinking coffee out of a little silver filigree cup and smoking a diamond-covered pipe, and "sitting up all night in the ladies cabin of a ship, nine to the square yard," with screaming children who were covered in fleas. Years later, when planning the arrangements for sending Nightingale nurses to Australia, she commented, "When I think of what kind of women I have slept with (twenty in the same cabin and all over the floor)," she felt anyone who had to share a cabin with the nice, clean Nightingale nurses was lucky.[29]

But if Nightingale was well educated in nursing and Eastern living conditions when she landed at Scutari, she was not educated in the political maneuvering that became necessary as she and the War Office, not all of whose members were supportive of her assignment,[30] worked with an army medical department which had not asked for her help and which resented her arrival.

Nightingale's Challenges in the East

Working with the Doctors

Nightingale arrived in Scutari on 4 November 1854. The medical officers would not allow her nurses in the hospitals, and the purveyors would not give her hospital stores and clothing. However, before the end of the first week she had succeeded in gaining entrance to the two Scutari hospitals for some of her nurses. On 9 November crowds of wounded soldiers in the worst stages of destitution began to arrive after the battle of Inkerman on 5 November. The nurses then became more welcome, but even so, Nightingale wrote later, referring to the entire war, "the number of nurses admitted into each division of a hospital depended on the medical officer of that division, who sometimes accepted them, sometimes refused them, sometimes accepted them after they had been refused; while the duties they were permitted to perform varied according to the will of each individual medical officer."[31]

Three illustrations suffice to demonstrate how Nightingale aligned herself with the medical men. Many hospital nurses showed a grievous lack of discipline, drinking too much, failing to come to work, or coming late, and once in the wards, not doing the work and failing to follow medical orders. As well, the social behavior of many did not meet middle-class standards of respectability. Nightingale knew that if her team contravened the strict Victorian rules of propriety, her venture would become a travesty, a repeat of the earlier experiments mentioned by the Duke of Newcastle, and she therefore ferociously insisted on strict obedience to her orders. In the contract she wrote for the nurses she made their three worst failings—neglect of duty, immoral conduct, and drunkenness—cause for dismissal.[32]

The six St. John's House nurses had none of these weaknesses. Yet in December 1854 Nightingale began arranging to dismiss four of them because, she said, they were inexperienced nurses and did not follow the rules. They went into the wards at night alone, which she forbade, and worst of all, fed the men without medical orders.[33] Three of the six St. John's House nurses were indeed relatively inexperienced. One had less than a year's experience, and two began their training in the summer of 1854.[34] Nevertheless, three months' training was a long period of training in 1854, and these women considered themselves trained nurses. As well, having been trained by a sisterhood, they were used to being treated with respect. "We do not look for many comforts," Elizabeth Drake wrote the lady superintendent in December 1854, "but we do feel we ought to be trusted. We are not allowed to go into the wards without one of the lady nurses. We must not speak one word of comfort to a poor dying man or read to him. We are prevented from doing what our hearts prompt us to do. We feel we are not so useful as we expected to be."[35]

These nurses could not understand Nightingale's draconian insistence that doctors' orders be literally obeyed because they conflicted with the supportive treatment in which they had been trained. But no matter how the feverish men might beg for a drink, if the medical men had not ordered fluids, Nightingale would not allow the nurses to provide them. She did not want the nurses speaking or reading to the men, for two reasons: she feared that they might establish personal relationships and that they might read sectarian literature, which could give rise to religious disputes.[36] But above all, Nightingale would not tolerate nurses acting without doctors' orders; she dismissed them summarily when they did. Later, when she felt her position better established, she would treat the working-class women more kindly.[37]

The problem with Sister Elizabeth Wheeler, one of the Devonport Sisters of Mercy, was of a different nature. Wheeler was anxious to feed her patients everything the doctors ordered, and at the end of November, when supplies were especially limited, she annoyed everyone by seeking preferential treatment for her patients.[38] Then she sent a letter to a relative asking him to send wine, chicken broth, preserved meats, and other food that shipped well. The relative sent the letter to *The Times*, which published it on 8 December 1854.[39] Sister Elizabeth's letter appears innocuous to the modern reader, but because it was made public and indicated failure on the part of the government and the army's medical department and supply system, Nightingale supported the doctors in ruthlessly dismissing her, even testifying against her.

A commission of three doctors and a lawyer examined Wheeler on 23 December, trying to get her to admit that her letter was inaccurate. They did not give her a copy of her letter and did not tell her which statements they considered untrue. Wheeler was wholly unprepared for the trial and became confused and appeared to prevaricate. The doctors pronounced her letter contradictory to her verbal evidence and tried to make her admit that she had lied. They threatened her with penal consequences if she did not sign the confession they had written, but Wheeler refused to sign, saying she was not aware she had told any untruth. The commission decided she must be dismissed immediately, and the next morning, Christmas Eve, Nightingale fired her.[40] Nightingale was in Scutari to nurse the soldiers, but she was also there with her team of nurses to appease the public outcry over the lack of supplies and medical care, and Wheeler's letter fed that outcry.

In October 1855 Charles Bracebridge, now back in England, gave a lecture severely criticizing the army doctors' medical treatment of the men and claiming that most of the improvements in the hospitals were Nightingale's work. *The Times* published the lecture, enraging the doctors. Nightingale thought they were justly provoked and sent Bracebridge a sharp letter of reproof. His statements about the doctors were utterly untrue, she said, and even if they were true, it was not his business to say so. They were unfair and justified the accusations that the nurses meddled in medical therapeutics. They exposed her to accusations of feminine interference when she was most anxious to avoid what might be called women's quarrels. Worse, such statements lessened her influence and seemed to place her in an adversarial stance vis-à-vis the doctors.[41] Nightingale thought that after such a lecture Bracebridge could not return to the East; if he did, he would greatly injure her work. In any case, she found it easier without him. She thought that if a woman did not shock the officers' "business habits or their caste prejudices," they would extend courtesy to her, something they would not do to a man who, as Bracebridge had, pitted the civilians against the military and the nurses against the doctors.[42] This was one of the few instances in which she found a certain advantage in being female.

Working with the Ladies

Nightingale did not think highly of most of her secular lady nurses. She would later write that "volunteer untrained ladies offering themselves for war and emergencies" were the "greatest mischief of all in her experience."[43] Some of the ladies refused to accept her supervision, for as Anne Summers points out, ladies in Victorian England were subordinate to their male relatives in law, but in the domestic sphere—in their own homes and in their charitable activities—they were far more used to giving orders than to taking them.[44] Ladies such as Martha Clough and Margaret Wear, both of whom had the advantage of being posted in the Crimea, far away from Scutari, enjoyed evading Nightingale's control.

When Clough left the Balaclava General Hospital to which Nightingale had assigned her and took over Sir Colin Campbell's regimental hospital, Nightingale wrote asking for an explanation. "I very coolly wrote back to her," Clough told a friend, "telling her that as I did not consider myself accountable to her, I declined giving her my reasons, that I acknowledged no authority here but that of Lord Raglan [the commander-in-chief of the British army in the East], and Sir Colin Campbell, and at home the Secretary at War." Clough believed she had the full support of Lord Stratford de Redcliffe, the ambassador to Turkey, as well and thought she was indeed "a match for Nightingale." She concluded, "So I think the Nightingale will have a tough job to un-nest me."[45]

Margaret Wear, for some months lady superintendent of the Balaclava General Hospital, was another lady who wished to work independently of Nightingale. She had the support of Sir John Hall, the principal medical officer in the East, and would cause Nightingale much grief colluding with him to reject her authority. She told Hall in October 1855 that she considered Nightingale to have released her from all obligation to her and to her orders, something that Nightingale had not done. From now on, Wear said, she was completely at Hall's disposal and would obey his orders only.[46]

Nightingale's friend Mary Stanley was yet another lady who rejected her authority. In early December 1854 Nightingale learned that Stanley was sailing from England with a large group of ladies, Roman Catholic nuns, and hospital nurses. Nightingale wrote Herbert, objecting strongly to the additional women. Dr. Menzies, the chief medical officer at the Scutari hospitals, believed there were already as many nurses in the two hospitals as could, "with morality and discipline," be properly employed. Nightingale fully agreed with him and said she would resign if she were forced to accept this new party. "The discipline of 40 women collected together for the first time," she wrote, "is no trifling matter under these new and strange circumstances." If the number were increased to 60 or 70, good order would become impossible. There were actually 46 women in Stanley's party, who together with Nightingale's original group made a total of 84.[47]

In addition to the doctors' orders and the disciplinary problem, it was impossible to house such a large group in the two hospitals. In order to maintain discipline Nightingale felt it essential to have the women under her eye. Moving more women into the already overcrowded nurses' quarters would be unhealthy and would mean Nightingale would have to spend more energy on governing the women than nursing the soldiers. The soldiers were laid up to the door of the few rooms assigned to the nurses in the Barrack Hospital, and Nightingale had given some of the exiguous space assigned to the nurses in the General Hospital to the patients. In the Barrack Hospital the rain poured into every room in the nurses' quarters, and there were no houses in Scutari suitable for Englishwomen. Furthermore, the nurses were sometimes without food or charcoal. Those who worked in the General Hospital lived in the Barrack Hospital and had to walk about a half mile to and from the hospital twice each day. They could not move into the hospital until a stove was installed, and all the available workmen were busy repairing the sick wards, to which Nightingale gave priority. All these factors, Nightingale said, demonstrated the difficulty of having more women and especially ladies in Scutari.[48]

Mary Stanley and her party had already sailed when Nightingale was writing Herbert. On their arrival in Turkey on 15 December, Stanley claimed that Herbert had assigned her party not to Nightingale but to Dr. Cumming, the principal medical officer of the Barrack Hospital, a statement Herbert later denied. Nightingale was furious. She told Stanley she was resigning and asked Stanley to succeed her at once. Stanley had the good sense to refuse.[49] As there was no space for the new women in the two Scutari hospitals, they were quartered elsewhere.

Nightingale sent Herbert another irate letter, pointing out, among other things, that there was an excessive number of Roman Catholics in the Stanley party—Mother Francis Bridgeman and her fourteen nuns.[50] Sue Goldie and Mark Bostridge suggest that had Nightingale been more gracious about accepting these nuns, she might have avoided the later struggle with Bridgeman,[51] but Nightingale's orders did not give her this option, and throughout the war she followed the War Office's instructions to the letter. She was extraordinarily consistent where principles were concerned, despite Monica Baly's frequently quoted statement that she was nothing if not inconsistent. More to the point is Hugh Small's comment that if anything Nightingale was too rational; far from being very complicated, she may be one of the easiest persons to understand once one recognizes what she was trying to accomplish.[52]

Nightingale had ten nuns already in the hospitals, which was causing an outcry, and she had to keep the number of Roman Catholics in any single hospital at a ratio of one to three. "I have toiled my way into the confidence of the medical men," she told Herbert, and "by incessant vigilance day and night, introduced something like system into the disorderly operations of these women." Dr. Menzies would allow only two more Roman Catholics in the General Hospital, and Nightingale could not add any more at the Barrack Hospital "without exciting the suspicion of the medical men and others." The doctors had set fifty nurses of any denomination as the maximum number they would accept in the two hospitals, and Nightingale, in line with her policy of always supporting the medical men, completely agreed with this figure.[53]

Nightingale told Herbert she had followed his orders in as consistent a manner as possible under extremely difficult conditions. She reiterated his instructions: "(1) Establish no separate action from the medical men but be their lieutenant and purveyor to carry out their intentions. (2) Control among your charge all these different sects and views so as to prevent these hospitals from becoming a 'polemical arena'—I quote your own words." Stanley's party made it almost impossible to implement these directions. These ladies saw their job as a religious, not a nursing, mission. Stanley wanted ten Roman Catholic nuns to act as assistants to the priests and ten Protestant ladies as assistants to the chaplains.[54]

It was no accident that Stanley's group had a high proportion of Roman Catholics, for Stanley was in fact, if not in name, a member of the Roman Catholic party. Nightingale was fully aware that Stanley had been consulting Dr. Manning about converting to Catholicism well before her trip to Scutari. Her brother, an Anglican cleric, had asked Nightingale to try to prevent her conversion. And indeed, while in the East, Stanley did finally convert. When Nightingale and Cumming did not give her government money, Stanley applied to Lord Stratford for funding.[55] Further complicating the sensitive religious issue, placing Stanley under Cumming with funding from the ambassador seemed to set up a second nursing team with a decidedly Roman Catholic coloration.

The Political Problem

Anti-Catholicism and the Papal Aggression

Why did Nightingale, Herbert, and the doctors think it so important to keep the number of Roman Catholics low? The flood of impoverished Irish laborers into England in the first part of the nineteenth century intensified the long tradition of anti-Catholicism, which was shared by all social classes. This influx reached its peak during the years of the famine after 1845. Unskilled Roman Catholic Irish laborers were prepared to accept the lowest wages and tended to congregate in destitute quarters, where their religion, social habits, and poverty made them difficult to assimilate. The flood of cheap Irish labor depressed the Protestant labor market, and the displaced English workers identified Roman Catholicism with the Irish laborers who had taken their jobs from them.

Many Protestants thought Roman Catholics superstitious, morally corrupt, and a challenge to the Protestant Constitution. The history of two armed invasions of England (1715 and 1745) intended to overthrow the Protestant government and reinstate a Roman Catholic king fed Protestant fears. As well, many Protestants associated Roman Catholics with sexual depravity and absolute monarchies. The defeat of the Spanish Armada in 1588, seen as the victory of righteous Protestant sea power over a Roman Catholic tyranny, was part of the national mystique. There was a vast outpouring of vulgar "No Popery" literature, describing all kinds of sexual, and sometimes sexually deviant, relationships between nuns and priests, nuns being entombed live in their convents, and so on. Many pamphlets of this genre, based largely on prurient imagination and ignorance of the real tenets of Roman Catholicism,[56] were sent to the East during the war. Sister Mary Aloysius Doyle, one of the Bridgeman party and certainly no prude, thought these tracts with their horrible pictures so bad that she would not describe them. She burned thousands of them, believing she was doing as great a service to the Protestant soldiers as to the Catholic,[57] and she probably was.

The larger question of how Ireland was to be governed brought these issues into the center of English political life. In a society in which violence was endemic, there were anti-Catholic disturbances from the Gordon Riots of 1780 on throughout the nineteenth century. The governing classes of Britain were obsessed with what they considered the Popish menace. The number of governments that fell because of the Irish question, beginning with Pitt's ministry in 1801, was very large.[58] Then, in 1850, there was an exceptionally acute resurgence of anti-Catholic feeling. Since the Reformation, Roman Catholic parishes in Britain were treated as missions; they were governed by four vicars apostolic. In 1840, because of the large immigration of Irish Roman Catholics, the pope increased the number of vicars apostolic to eight, and in 1850, he established twelve bishoprics, something which had not existed in England since the sixteenth century, and made the militant Irishman Nicholas Wiseman a cardinal and the archbishop of Westminster, a title that infuriated many

Englishmen, including Lord John Russell, the prime minister. Wiseman thought England was on the threshold of a massive return to what he and other Roman Catholics considered the true faith, an event he personally hoped to help effect.[59]

The creation of the Roman Catholic bishoprics caused a massive popular upheaval and crisis known as the Papal Aggression. It resulted in a new wave of violent anti-Catholicism and also aroused vicious controversies among the Dissenting denominations and within the established church itself. From the late 1830s religious tensions had been increasing among the Protestant denominations over the issues of church rates and denominational education. The established church encompassed three major movements: the High Church party, which stressed continuity with the pre-Reformation church; the Broad Church party, which wished to be all-inclusive; and the Low Church or Evangelical party. Because many identified it with popery, the High Church or Anglo-Catholic party suffered the most fierce attacks and opposition, and Low Churchmen and Dissenters often formed alliances against it.[60] The Park Village and Devonport Sisters of Mercy, temporarily under the direction of Mother Priscilla Lydia Sellon, were very High Church. In an effort to disassociate herself from the much maligned and disliked position of the High Church, Nightingale thought it politically wise to call these sisters Sellonites and to refer to Miss Wheeler rather than to Sister Elizabeth, so that people would not confuse Anglican sisters with the Roman Catholic Sisters of Mercy. However, no one else used this term.

The importance of the Irish question and the government's dependence on the Irish vote in Parliament weighed heavily on Nightingale. "We are afraid of the Roman Catholics," she bemoaned. "If a man is a Roman Catholic, the government will say, 'Oh! Do pray be quiet, don't tell us of his lies or you will bring the Roman Catholics down upon us.'" But much as she would have liked to, she knew it was politically impossible to send the Stanley party home. She started incorporating Stanley's nurses, and by the end of January, with the exception of those who had been dismissed or left, had placed all of them in the hospitals in Scutari, Koulali, and Balaclava.[61]

After the Bracebridges sailed for home at the end of July 1855,[62] Stanley's worst characteristics came to the fore in the notorious Salisbury case. Charlotte Salisbury, a former governess, had been hired to take over Selina Bracebridge's position as administrator of the Free Gift Store.[63] Salisbury began stealing and distributing the stores to her friends and even purloined some of Nightingale's clothes. Dismissed by Nightingale on 27 September, she returned to England, where she protested her innocence and, with the support of Mary Stanley and others, brought a widely advertised libel suit against Nightingale. This group enlisted the help of disgruntled war nurses, largely ones whom Nightingale had fired, to give evidence against her. At one point in February 1856 Nightingale expected that sixty-four charges of libel would be laid against her. The War Department investigated, found the charges untrue, and the action failed.[64]

Mother Francis Bridgeman: Irish Roman Catholic Militancy

Wear, Clough, and Stanley caused Nightingale difficulties, but from the government's point of view, these ladies were of little significance. By contrast, the Roman Catholic issue and its fundamental relationship to the Irish question was of immense political importance, and Mother Francis Bridgeman's aggressive refusal to cooperate with Nightingale would prove an insoluble problem. On first meeting with Nightingale in December 1854, Bridgeman quite understandably wanted to start work immediately but insisted that her party remain whole and under her direction. This was in accordance with the instructions of her bishop, Thomas Delany of Cork,[65] but it was obviously impossible under the circumstances. Bridgeman was unaware of Nightingale's orders from the War Office concerning the ratio of Roman Catholic nurses, and she did not take in the difficulty Nightingale had getting any nurses, much less Roman Catholic nuns, admitted to the hospitals. Mother Mary Clare Moore thought Bridgeman and her sisters did not completely understand the situation. Although Bridgeman had signed the contract with the government agreeing to serve under Nightingale,[66] Moore wrote, she and her nuns "refused on reaching Constantinople to be subject to Miss Nightingale. They had the idea that they might hire a house in the town of Scutari, form a regular religious community and attend the hospitals as they could have done in Ireland."[67]

Nightingale's interpretation that Bridgeman had come out "with a religious view, not to serve the sick but to found a convent," was not quite accurate but was not far off. Bridgeman and her sisters were excellent, experienced nurses who did indeed serve the sick well, but for them "mere nurse-tending," as Bishop Delany put it, took second place to what they considered the higher end of saving souls, something Nightingale was wary of because Herbert had prohibited the nurses from proselytizing.[68]

Nightingale and Bridgeman shared many characteristics. Both were deeply religious; both were fine, experienced administrators who appreciated the importance of undivided authority; and both were excellent, experienced nurses.[69] Both were committed to nursing soldiers of any faith, and both were truthful—their accounts of their various meetings support each other in every detail. However, the two women took an immediate personal dislike to each other[70] and differed strongly in their approach to sectarianism. Nightingale was probably one of the few ladies in England who was prepared to accept Roman Catholics on an equal footing. Two of her best friends before the war were Roman Catholics, Mother Santa Columba in Rome and Dr. Manning. Mother Mary Clare Moore became her greatest support during the war and one of her closest friends.[71] Bridgeman was an accomplished and highly competent lady, much respected by her nuns,[72] but she was also a product of centuries of brutal English oppression in Ireland. Her strong Irish nationalism and anti-English prejudice led her to consider Nightingale "an insidious, dangerous enemy," propped up "by human power and English infatuation and bigotry." She thought no one who knew Nightingale could trust her: she was ill-mannered and dishonest, the doctors generally disliked her, and the success of Bridgeman's sisters keenly excited her jealousy. She believed Nightingale's nursing service had no system and the only nurses in the East who could be relied on were her own nuns. Finally, she thought Nightingale opposed her at every turn and wished her to resign,[73] which was not true.

Bridgeman's fervent anti-English bias induced her to be misled by false tales and rumors. The departure of the five Norwood nuns is a good example of her gullibility. These nuns had little experience nursing the sick and their white habits were so impractical that Nightingale decided to send them home and replace them with five of Bridgeman's sisters.[74] Bridgeman was not in Scutari when the Norwood nuns left, but she repeated a story that Nightingale had dismissed them "on very short notice and in the *most humiliating manner.* Together with some nurses dismissed for bad conduct she marched them through the hospital in their white habits to the main gate where she called out their names and formally dismissed them." Even their enemies, Bridgeman wrote, said the Norwood nuns were not incompetent: Nightingale discharged them because she disliked their habits. In fact, Vicar General Robert Whitty of Westminster told Moore that he had visited the Norwood nuns after their return home and that they spoke most kindly of Nightingale. "Not a word of complaint has come from them," he said, but the same could not be said of their friends in the world. There was a great deal of criticism and complaint about the treatment of the nuns in the Roman Catholic papers, which Whitty regretted.[75]

The Politics of Gender: Sir John Hall and Feminine Interference

Bridgeman became a natural ally of Sir John Hall, the officer to whom Nightingale ultimately reported and whom she considered her most formidable enemy.[76] In the *Dictionary of National Biography* Mark Harrison treats Hall very favorably, describing him as a hard worker and an able, courageous, and efficient officer. Nightingale herself called him an able and efficient officer, although she added that he was good at details but incapable of governing. Born in 1795, Hall campaigned against Napoleon in Flanders in 1815, and during the Crimean War he was personally on the scene of many engagements. In Bombay, just before coming to the Crimea, he instituted reforms in medical statistics and barrack accommodation. Trained at Guy's and St. Thomas' hospitals, he was a Fellow of the Royal College of Surgeons. Harrison believes that his contemporaries in Britain and overseas held Hall in the highest regard.[77] But Hall was unhappy from the beginning with what he considered the newspapers' exaggerated reports of the lack of medical care, he resented the intrusion of The Times Fund,[78] and he was adamantly opposed to Nightingale. Goldie points out that it was largely the older doctors, veterans of the Napoleonic wars, who did not accept Nightingale, while her principal supporters were younger doctors. Herbert thought Hall considered efforts to offer assistance "slurs on his preparations." "The exaggerated attacks of *The Times* make him take refuge in secrecy," Herbert wrote, "instead of meeting them by exertions to remedy deficiencies."[79]

Hall's dealings with Nightingale were clearly not his finest hour. He "descends to every meanness to make my position more difficult," she wrote her Aunt Mai in October 1855. He took advantage of a loophole in her appointment which placed her in charge of the nursing in Turkey and did not mention Russia. Lord Raglan, of course, had asked her to send nurses to the Crimea, but Hall asserted, though he denied it to Nightingale, that she had no authority beyond Turkey. Nightingale believed he promised the nurses in the Crimea that if they would desert her, he would pay their wages.[80]

When Mary Stanley went home at the beginning of April 1855, Nightingale resigned as superintendent of the Koulali Hospitals. Unable to elicit cooperation from the Koulali nurses, who were largely directed by Bridgeman, she wanted to "be in no way responsible for the conduct and expenditure of those sisters."[81] After Nightingale resigned, Bridgeman was supposed to report to General Storks, the commander of the British Establishment in Turkey. In April 1855, when the Castle Hospital opened, Raglan decided to keep the wounded in Balaclava and sent only convalescents to Turkey, where they were concentrated in the Scutari hospitals. As a result there was little work in Koulali, and at the beginning of September, without consulting Storks, Bridgeman offered to take her nuns to Balaclava to work directly under Hall. Hall jumped at this opportunity to rid the Balaclava General Hospital of Nightingale. Referring to a letter of 14 July 1855 in which Nightingale said she was short-staffed and would like to withdraw her nurses from that hospital until at least October, and without telling her of Bridgeman's offer, Hall asked Nightingale to recall her nurses. Nightingale agreed to do so and wrote Wear accordingly.[82] Wear immediately sent the letter to Hall. Wear, Hall, and purveyor David Fitzgerald, an Irish Roman Catholic who supported Hall's efforts to thwart Nightingale, exchanged Nightingale's letters and their replies, frequently making hostile comments on them.[83]

Hall stayed correctly within military regulations in his dealings with Nightingale, but Fitzgerald was less restrained. He was a difficult person, and Nightingale was by no means the only one to have problems working with him. Dr. Beatson, the head doctor at the Balaclava General Hospital, forbade him to interfere in the internal arrangements of the hospital and told the attendants not to take orders from him. Dr. Mouat, who was in charge of the field hospitals at Sevastopol, actually had Fitzgerald arrested for what he termed his capriciousness and "independent authority." Fitzgerald would question a requisition on the grounds of the spelling of a word. Mouat commented sarcastically that Fitzgerald was not a philologist, much less competent "to make impertinent comments thereon." Yet Hall supported Fitzgerald. At the end of December 1855 Fitzgerald sent a "Confidential Report" on the nursing to the War Department. This report extolled Bridgeman's nuns and was devastatingly critical of Nightingale's nurses. Nightingale privately obtained a copy almost immediately.[84]

Nightingale first learned of Bridgeman's new appointment in October 1855, when Bridgeman informed her that together with her Koulali nuns she was taking her sisters who were then working in the Scutari hospitals to Balaclava. Nightingale consulted General Storks and the ambassador, both of whom told her she would be fully within her rights if she were to stop them from going. She decided against that course because she did not wish to create a breach between Roman Catholics and Protestants.[85] Instead, in an effort to maintain the integrity of the team, she accompanied Bridgeman to the Crimea. On the surface Nightingale maintained friendly relations with her, but she told Charles Bracebridge that Bridgeman's conduct was "neither that of a Christian, a gentlewoman nor even of a woman." Nevertheless, Nightingale said, she was prepared to do or submit to anything "to avoid a woman's quarrel."[86]

The party arrived in Balaclava on 13 October 1855, and the following day Nightingale had a lengthy interview with Hall. She explained the required one-to-three ratio for Roman Catholics, and Hall agreed that no further nurses should be admitted to the hospitals in the East without her knowledge and consent. Hall claimed Nightingale had quoted instructions that were previously unknown to him.[87] But were they? Sir Benjamin Hawes, under-secretary for war and not generally supportive of Nightingale, claimed that Hall had been officially informed of Nightingale's position as superintendent of the ladies and nurses in the East,[88] and Hall certainly knew that Raglan had invited her nurses to the Crimea and that he considered them under her authority.

By November 1855 Nightingale felt that Hall was no longer concealing his efforts to force her out of the Crimea "by petty pricks." In July 1855 he had told Nightingale, who had been very ill, that she would have recovered far sooner if she had left Turkey, and now he told her the Crimean climate was bad for her. In compliance with her instructions to strictly obey the purveyors, Nightingale's superintendents never issued any food or clothing without a requisition from the doctor in charge. At Balaclava, Hall insisted on adhering strictly to a regulation that he himself must personally countersign each requisition as well as the attending doctor. Nightingale called him "the prince of red tape and inhuman routine."[89]

When the Monastery Hospital opened and Hall appointed Wear superintendent, Nightingale thought it best to go along with it rather than lose control of the hospital. The Smyrna hospital was closing, and Fitzgerald, without consulting Nightingale, wrote to its lady superintendent, Miss LeMesurier, asking her to send two of her nurses to the Monastery Hospital.[90] LeMesurier sent the two via Scutari, where Nightingale kept them and sent different nurses to Wear. Wear wrote Hall that Nightingale had better not send any more of her people unless Hall wished it. Despite the fact that he had agreed no nurses would be transferred in or out of hospitals without Nightingale's knowledge, Hall encouraged Wear, replying that he did not understand Nightingale's actions—he could not see why Nightingale had not sent the Smyrna nurses to the Monastery.[91]

"Few persons in England could understand how greatly Miss Nightingale was opposed all throughout her efforts to improve the military hospital system," Mother Mary Clare Moore wrote. She thought the opposition reached its climax in the Crimea.[92] Nightingale's modern critics have been less generous. Winfried Baumgart characterizes her as "imperious and haughty" when dealing with nurses, doctors, and bureaucrats. Martha Vicinus, Bea Nergaard, and Goldie think Nightingale was arrogant and showed a remarkable lack of tact and magnanimity in her dealings with Hall. Her letters, in their opinion, did not jibe with the protestations of humility and obedience to the medical officers which she frequently made. Goldie believes Nightingale could have avoided the struggle with Hall.[93] Nightingale could be high-handed, as when she dismissed the St. John's House nurses, but Gillian Gill points out that it was only in her letters to her friends and family that Nightingale expressed herself unreservedly. Gill characterizes her direct dealings with Hall as "suave and diplomatic,"[94] and it is worth noting that Nightingale never once disobeyed Hall's orders.

Nightingale went back to Scutari at the end of November 1855 because of a cholera outbreak but returned to the Crimea in March 1856 to take on the nursing of the two Land Transport hospitals at the invitation of their principal medical officer, Dr. George Taylor. The preceding month, in response to her request, the War Office issued a General Order stating that Nightingale was general superintendent of all the army's hospitals and that no nurse was to be transferred from one hospital to another or introduced without consulting her. This order was published in Sevastopol on 16 March 1856.[95] Armed with this clear definition of her authority, Nightingale hoped to find her job easier when she met with Bridgeman; in fact, it would cause Bridgeman to resign. Having all Roman Catholic nurses in one hospital was entirely contrary to her original instructions from the War Office, but, Nightingale wrote, "in this instance, common prudence and feeling" dictated leaving them there. "I shall interfere with them in no way whatever," she told Col. Lefroy, her friend in the War Office, for she was afraid the nuns might resign and thereby make martyrs of themselves.[96]

Nightingale arrived in Balaclava on 24 March and the next day went to see Bridgeman. She informed Bridgeman that Dr. Beatson had told her how much he valued her nuns. She knew the General Order caused Bridgeman uneasiness, and to set her mind at ease Nightingale committed to not interfering or making any change so long as Dr. Hall was satisfied. Bridgeman would not accept this arrangement and responded, "Thank you, Miss Nightingale, but to admit to an authority and to submit to it is one and the same thing with us. I shall not place myself and sisters in such a false position as to admit your right of superintendence and then restrict it or refuse to submit to it." Nightingale reminded her that she had signed a contract agreeing to work under her direction. Bridgeman replied that while she had originally planned to do so, experience had taught her better. Referring to Nightingale's refusal to accept her whole party at Scutari in December 1854, she told her, "You refused us. You yourself dissolved the connection."[97]

"I have had a curious breeze with Mrs. Bridgeman," Nightingale wrote her Aunt Mai, "which for abominable hypocrisy and astuteness on the part of that woman beats the world." On the other hand, Nightingale and Fitzgerald "met like the oldest friends. But he knows," Nightingale said, that "I know 'it' [i.e., the Confidential Report]. We are obliged to have hourly business together in his office and he will shoot me if he can." Although she was able to work with Fitzgerald, Nightingale was unable to work out a modus vivendi with Bridgeman. Bridgeman said she was willing to submit to any sacrifice or humiliation but she would resign rather than nominally work under Nightingale. One of Bridgeman's nuns, Sister Joseph Croke, illustrated the impossibility of compromise when she wrote that Nightingale was "struck down" when she saw "Rev. Mother's determination not to recognize her authority, now that Dr. Hall has exercised his faculties and absolved her from subjection [to Nightingale]." Croke thought Nightingale "crestfallen since the Sisters of Mercy had escaped her fangs."[98]

In her final interview with Bridgeman, when Nightingale at last realized that nothing could make her change her mind, Bridgeman said Nightingale became quite hysterical. "She laughed hysterically," Bridgeman wrote, and "used the most groundless and contradictory arguments. She said Revd. Mother [Bridgeman] was putting a stone of stumbling between the churches, which she was trying to remove." Bridgeman believed Nightingale had constantly put obstacles in her path and laughed at Nightingale's statement. "Miss Nightingale raised her hand," she wrote: "and shaking it at Revd Mother she exclaimed as one might to a naughty school child, 'Don't laugh, don't laugh.' She really quite frightened Revd. Mother....When they were shaking hands parting, while shaking Revd. Mother's hands, most emphatically, she was exclaiming, 'God forgive you, God forgive you.'" Nightingale told Bridgeman that she would always remember that day as the worst day in her life, the day she would most regret.[99]

For a woman who was noted for always maintaining a calm, lady-like exterior, Nightingale's loss of composure is an indication of how much it meant to her to have given up hope of any kind of cooperation with Bridgeman's contingent. "I so deeply regret that the General Order should have produced this consequence," she wrote Lefroy. "I can only add that I thought most seriously of resigning the General Hospital at Balaclava for the sake of peace." But it would have been impossible to preserve discipline or morality among the nurses, she said, if she resigned when they rebelled, nor could she have one rule for Roman Catholics and another for Anglicans.[100]

An Important Lesson in Political Skills

Nightingale wrote a detailed refutation of Fitzgerald's Confidential Report, which is well supported by other sources. Fitzgerald made numerous errors of fact as well as of interpretation. For example, he claimed that in July 1855 five of the eleven nurses at the Castle and General hospitals, Mrs. Davies, Sandhouse, Lawfield, Noble, and Tuffill, were dismissed for insubordination, violence, or irregular conduct. Mrs. Davies, Mrs. Noble, and Mrs. Tuffill were invalided home on the advice of Drs. Hall and Anderson, their health broken "by their unremitting devotion to their duty," as Nightingale put it. Fitzgerald himself had publicly said that Mrs. Davies ought to receive a pension from government; she was worth twice the wages. Mrs. Lawfield was still in Balaclava and was a woman of faultless character. Mrs. Sandhouse was sent home not because of any failing in character but because she was not an efficient nurse. Nightingale's anger flames throughout her refutation of Fitzgerald's report. She called it "a tissue of unfounded assertions, wilful perversions and, in some instances, malicious and scandalous libels." If she had not felt it necessary to clear the reputation of nurses who were unjustly and secretly accused, she said, she would not have waded through "the filth cast upon them."[101]

In her fury Nightingale wrote Herbert requesting him to ask in the House of Commons to have her original instructions, the Confidential Report, and her refutation published. Herbert was no longer in the government but of course still sat in the House of Commons. A man of great personal charm and extraordinarily good temper, he had been closely associated with senior statesmen from his childhood. He had a keen sense of what was politically possible and efficacious,[102] and he was therefore very much against moving for the production of these papers in Parliament. In a long letter to Nightingale, Herbert told her, "It will always be time to produce papers in your vindication when you are attacked, and so long as there is no public attack on you, you stand better than you would if publicly attacked and triumphantly defended."[103]

Making the Confidential Report public would show, Herbert said, that Hall questioned the competence of Nightingale's nurses, and Roman Catholics would accept his belief in the superiority of Bridgeman's nuns as true. The Salisbury and Stanley parties would take up the Hall and Fitzgerald views and press their case, and the public would think that "it was a pack of women quarreling among themselves." If Hall and Fitzgerald published or moved in Parliament for the production of the report, it would be time enough for Nightingale to defend her position.

Finally, Herbert thought Nightingale was overrating the importance of Fitzgerald's report. She was forgetting that she held an official government position. The vehemence and irritation with which she responded detracted from the weight that would otherwise attach to what she said. "I see in Fitzgerald's report," he wrote, "nothing more than the unfair, biased, special pleading report of a narrow-minded religionist. These are misrepresentations and annoyances which all persons in office, and you are in office, are exposed to."

He urged her not to characterize but rather to disprove Fitzgerald's statements. If she did so in a calm way, the reader would be more likely to accept her accuracy. He cited the McNeill-Tulloch Report on the supply system of the army as an example of the right tone—"not a hard word in it," he said, "or an epithet, not an accusation, scarcely an animadversion." It was always wise, he advised, "in a public document to understate your case. If on examination your case proves stronger than you have stated it to be, you reap the whole advantage. If, however, any part, however slight, is shaken, the credit of the whole is shaken with it."

Herbert's advice made Nightingale even more furious. She replied in what has become one of her most famous letters. "I received your letter of 6 March yesterday. It is written from Belgrave Square, I write from a Crimean hut. The point of sight is different." He had a warm fire and good dinner every day while she was struggling to feed and warm her nurses. She then went on to challenge every point Herbert had made.[104] Later, in a calmer mood, she took his advice to heart. Nightingale was used to working against opposition and to making compromises, but it was in the Crimea that she learned to think strategically and to avoid publicly expressing her personal vehemence and irritation. She dropped her demand that her orders, the Confidential Report, and her refutation be produced in Parliament. Her *Notes on Matters Affecting the Health, Efficiency and Hospital Administration of the British Army*, written in 1857–58 and considered by many her finest work,[105] was composed in precisely the style Herbert recommended.

Conclusion

Nightingale's mission in the Crimean War is without doubt her best-known venture and is traditionally seen as the beginning of nursing reform in England. A century after her death and a century and a half after the Crimean War, her work in the military hospitals deserves revisiting. As Bostridge writes, Nightingale's withdrawal from public life two years after the war allowed the public to sentimentalize her as the compassionate, saintly, ministering angel whose shadow the soldiers kissed.[106] The much greater number of sources now available reveal a more complex picture of a lady who was indeed compassionate but who also had to navigate the political straits of working for the government and the army. In order to understand the difficult decisions she had to make, we must place Nightingale beyond the narrower context of nursing reform into a broader framework: the Victorian constraints on ladies which made exercising authority in a male organization so problematic, the complex interrelationships of Victorian religious sectarianism and politics, and the political nature of her mission. It is only then that we can see more accurately her weaknesses and her very real brilliance.

In the task of organizing care for the soldiers, a massive job in itself and a story beyond the scope of this chapter, three major factors, all deeply rooted in the social foundation of Victorian society, made Nightingale's job infinitely more complicated. First, she had to work with a very disparate group of women in what was normally a segregated society. The much acclaimed secular lady nurses, not all of whom were prepared to accept her authority, did not have the necessary experience or knowledge to nurse the soldiers whereas the religious sisters, who were excellent clinical nurses, were sources of the very controversies she had been ordered to prevent. The working-class nurses presented a different set of problems: many had real nursing expertise, but what Victorians considered respectability was not a part of their culture. Nevertheless, by the end of the war Nightingale had established a respectable and efficient nursing service.

Second, in order to run an efficient nursing service, Nightingale had to contravene the Victorian convention that ladies should not exercise authority in the public sphere. This social prohibition played into the hands of those doctors and purveyors who could not reconcile themselves to a government-appointed lady in their midst. Nightingale succeeded in working with Fitzgerald, although she knew he detested her. She did not win over all the doctors, but in Hall's case she successfully obtained a General Order confirming her authority in Russia. Deeply humiliated, Hall finally admitted defeat and acknowledged her official position.[107]

Nightingale's success with her nursing team and the majority of the doctors had wider ramifications than the Crimean War, for it made inroads into the Victorian trivialization of women's activities. Herbert appreciated that her political difficulties could be interpreted as a pack of women quarreling among themselves, and it is striking how many times Nightingale felt she had to act so as to prevent the accusation that she was indulging in "a woman's quarrel" or "feminine interference" when her real aim was to provide a good nursing service. She had to fight, as she put it, "the common opinion that the vanity, the gossip and the insubordination of women...make them unfit for and mischievous in the [army] service, however materially useful they may be in it." Many people believed nursing was "a silly display of feminine sensibilities," Nightingale wrote, but she considered it "a set of tools for the medical officers."[108] The Crimean War nurses went far in helping the much-looked-down-upon nurses gain respect. "We are the first women who have been suffered in the war-service," Nightingale wrote in 1856,[109] and in the sense that she and her nurses were accepted in the public sphere by most of the army doctors and purveyors, the government, and especially the public, Nightingale broke through a major gender barrier.

The third factor making Nightingale's position so challenging, the most difficult and the most politically sensitive, was navigating the straits of sectarian controversy. Nightingale worked well with Protestant nurses of all denominations and with the eight Roman Catholic nuns from Bermondsey.[110] However, she was defeated by Mother Francis Bridgeman's Irish nationalism and Roman Catholic militancy. After Nightingale told Bridgeman that she would not interfere in the running of the Balaclava General Hospital, it is difficult to see what more could have been done to appease her. Bridgeman came to the East determined to set up an independent religious community and succeeded in doing so in Koulali and in Balaclava until the General Order of 16 March 1856. She did leave four sisters in Scutari under Nightingale when she went to Koulali, but except for a few weeks at the Barrack Hospital in December 1854–January 1855, an arrangement that her colleague Mother Mary Clare Moore negotiated, Bridgeman herself worked independently of Nightingale throughout the war. For Bridgeman, it was wrong to place Roman Catholic religious under the direction of a secular, and especially a Protestant secular. After the war she thought it would be "little less than sinful presumption" to participate in another, similar venture.[111] Although Nightingale failed to prevent Bridgeman's resignation, in the end it did not cause the political uproar Nightingale had feared.

Nightingale was by no means wholly successful, but with the help of Sidney Herbert, she managed the political straits well and would later go on to become a consummate political lobbyist. At the beginning of the war the press made contradictory accusations that she was running a Roman Catholic, a Unitarian, a High Church Anglican, or a Low Church Anglican nursing service.[112] By 1855 these sectarian attacks ceased. Nightingale became a national heroine, and she and her nurses did a great deal to quell the public outcry over the care of the soldiers. Politically, her mission was a huge success, one of the few bright spots in a rather bungled war, but for Nightingale the nursing of the soldiers was the most important issue. Her own evaluation of the expedition was that the enormous publicity the nurses received damaged their relations with "our masters, the army surgeons." It excited hostility among some people, she said, and attracted some women who were only adventurers; some of the ladies and nurses rebelled, and others were often drunk. "Still, what we came to do has been done," she concluded. "The suffering to be relieved has been relieved."[113]

THE DREAM OF NURSING THE EMPIRE

JUDITH GODDEN*

Through the Nightingale Fund, Florence Nightingale sent two teams of nurses overseas. The first team went to Australia in response to a request by the New South Wales government for trained nurses. Lucy Osburn and five other nurses arrived in Sydney in March 1868 and were initially employed by the New South Wales government on a three-year contract.

By the time the Nightingale Fund sent the next team of nurses abroad, to Canada in 1875, Nightingale's hopes for Australian nursing had been shattered. She had refused to write to Lucy Osburn or the five other nurses anymore. Initially, she had thought of Australia as a land of promise, even one where she would find a refuge in her old age. By 1875 Australia was little more than a hellish pit that had destroyed her dreams and corrupted her nurses. No nurse was worse than Lucy Osburn, and few places worse than Sydney.

The nursing team sent to Canada in 1875 went on a very different basis than that of the Sydney team. It was sent as a personal favor to one of Nightingale's favorite lady superintendents, Maria Machin, who wished to return to her native Canada. Machin, like Osburn and so many

* I gratefully acknowledge the assistance of a Faculty Research Program grant from the Canadian High Commission for travel to Canada, and I thank Carol Helmstadter for valuable comments on a draft of this chapter.

other Nightingale matrons, encountered fierce and sustained opposition to her efforts to transform Montreal General Hospital. Three years later she gave up. She and her loyal nurses returned to England, having failed to implement Nightingale nursing in Canada. In this crisis, and after Machin's return to England, Nightingale was consistently and lovingly supportive, a superlative friend and mentor.

The experiences of the two overseas teams have been researched from the viewpoint of the two nursing superintendents.[1] In this chapter the two episodes are explored to better understand Florence Nightingale. Why did she reject Osburn, who is now honored as the founder of Nightingale nursing in Australia, but support Machin, who so clearly failed in this task in Canada? Four interconnected factors are key to understanding Nightingale's responses: the perceived suitability of the Nightingale Training School as an international model; her celebrity and the brittle basis on which it was founded; the extent to which the ventures reflected imperialist aims; and the impact of her isolated, bedridden lifestyle. What was this most celebrated invalid's view from her bed, and how did it constrain the effectiveness of her nursing school and her hopes for nursing the empire?

The Nightingale Fund

The Nightingale Training School for Nurses was established at St. Thomas' Hospital in 1860. It was financed by the Nightingale Fund, set up to recognize "the noble exertions of Miss Nightingale in the hospitals of the East." The idea of the fund was "to enable her, on her return to England, to establish a permanent institution for the training, sustenance and protection of nurses and to arrange for their proper instruction and employment in metropolitan hospitals."[2] It was an ideal in keeping with Nightingale's commitment, at least since her time at Harley Street, for nurses to have formal instruction.[3] Despite these good intentions, practical difficulties caused long-term problems.

From the beginning, Nightingale had serious reservations about the fund. When it was first proposed, she was fully occupied with caring for the casualties of the Crimean War and reluctant to commit herself to any future plans. Yet it was truly a once-only offer that was almost impossible for her to refuse. Nightingale did accept, but in terms that were "gracious but not enthusiastic." She responded that she was "very doubtful" if she would have sufficient "life and health for the work," but accepted "on the understanding of this great uncertainty and whether it will ever be possible for me to carry it out."[4]

Despite this dampening reply, the supporters of the fund enthusiastically raised money. Among their difficulties, two were particularly troublesome. One was sectarianism. In an age of bitter conflict between Roman Catholic and Protestant Christianity, both groups had promoted trained nursing, most notably the Evangelical deaconesses at Kaiserswerth in Germany, and the Irish Catholic orders of the Sisters of Charity and Sisters of Mercy.[5] The public would not support the Nightingale Fund if the nursing school was under the auspices of a religious rival. A second major difficulty was that Nightingale refused to commit herself to a fixed plan to spend the money. To ask her for a plan, she flatly stated, was reasonable only if she "had originally asked for the money, which of course I did not."[6]

The endemic religious conflict meant that the proposed school of nursing had to be nonsectarian, a tricky ideal, as Nightingale had discovered during the Crimean War. Nightingale could thus not establish the school under a religious sisterhood nor directly involve either of two dear friends who were in London and in a strong position to help. Most unusually for the time, and indicative of Nightingale's status and visionary genius, one friend headed an Anglican sisterhood and the other a Roman Catholic one: Sister Mary Jones, the superior of the Church of England sisterhood, St. John's House; and Mother Clare Moore, superior of the Sisters of Mercy at Bermondsey.[7] Reflecting her times, Nightingale found it unthinkable that women could work for the welfare of others without a religious motivation. It was also assumed that women worked for a salary only because of dire financial need: the ideal was voluntary philanthropic work, as undertaken by Nightingale during the Crimean War.[8] The solution was an ingenious amalgam of the altruistic motivation of religious orders and volunteer philanthropists with an insistence on the need to pay a salary in order to attract those who could undertake the hard physical work of nursing.

Once back in England, after the Crimean War ended, Nightingale still had no set plans for the Nightingale Fund. She had been seriously ill during the war, and in August 1857 suffered a collapse so severe that she was thought to be dying.[9] While the cause and extent of her collapse remains a matter of debate, her mental well-being was unlikely to have been assisted by her work at the time.[10] She had been preparing a statistical analysis of the mortality rates during the Crimean War, and it confirmed her worst fears. The deaths at Scutari and the other hospitals had fallen only after the implementation of (in Nightingale's words) "the excellent sanitary arrangements...introduced by the Sanitary Commission."[11] The Sanitary Commission had instituted public health measures four months after Nightingale had arrived in Turkey. Her statistics revealed that her base hospital at Scutari, with its appalling sanitation and overcrowding, had been by far the worst. There three in every eight patients had died. The figures revealed, as Hugh Small dramatically asserts, that "she had been running a death camp."[12]

For Nightingale and other Victorians, the concept of a "good death" was of central importance.[13] Nightingale was credited with providing physical and spiritual comfort as much as saving lives, as illustrated in Henry Longfellow's 1857 poem "Santa Filomena," with its famous line "A lady with a lamp." Nevertheless, there is little reason to doubt that her mortality statistics sickened Nightingale. Certainly, her war experience convinced her that effective nursing needed sanitary surroundings. Nightingale made reparation by dedicating herself to improving the appalling conditions of soldiers' lives. So dedicated was she that in what she imagined was her few remaining years—perhaps months—of life, she had little time to establish the proposed school of nursing.

The public had donated £44,039 to the Nightingale Fund which in contemporary purchasing power was over £3 million (more than US$5 million).[14] It was too large a sum to be ignored, and by 1860, four years later, the need for action was urgent. The original assumption was that Nightingale would head the new school herself, but it became clear that she was both unwilling and unable to do so. There were three main reasons for this: her illness, her celebrity, and her other commitments.

Much has been written about Nightingale's illness after the Crimean War and how she became a reclusive invalid. Like so many who nursed in wars, Nightingale had been severely ill and returned to England exhausted and traumatized. Even thirteen years later she described her war experience as "like a horrid spectre" at the back of her mind, "ever present, ready to spring out" on her.[15] The following year the horrors of the Franco-Prussian War rekindled her memories of admitting into hospitals "4,000 severely sick men in 17 days" and of their "dreadful frostbitten limbs, quite black, & with all the flesh fallen off as if they had been eaten by the White Ants."[16] Almost a decade after her 1857 collapse she repeatedly insisted that she was "entirely a prisoner to a couch," an overworked invalid too ill to visit other than family homes or to see any but the most essential visitors.[17] D. A. B. Young demonstrated that Nightingale's illness was almost certainly chronic brucellosis, an infection spread by drinking untreated milk. Its symptoms are highly variable and often intermittent but include fever, nausea, and painful inflammation of the spine.[18] Nightingale was prescribed drugs, including morphine, which helped to control the pain but could also account for her other symptoms such as episodes of retching.[19]

What is underestimated in many analyses about Nightingale's health is the effect of her lifestyle, especially during the decade after her 1857 breakdown. As she embraced the role of a terminally ill invalid, at least some of her mental and physical symptoms were exacerbated by lack of exercise.[20] The assumption that prolonged, extreme bed rest was essential for invalids dominated health care for at least another century. The tragedy was that Nightingale's lifestyle was in stark contrast to her robust common sense in her classic *Notes on Nursing*.

After the Crimean War, Nightingale's celebrity also caused her immense difficulty. The adulation of Nightingale was worldwide and unprecedented for a woman who was neither royal nor a religious leader: the nearest analogy is to imagine, in our own time, the public response if Princess Diana and Mother Teresa had been one person. The very modern problem of celebrity was compounded for Nightingale, as she was a private individual with no institutional power to protect her. As well, behavioral mores of the time meant that a "lady" eschewed publicity; such high-status women worked through influence, not direct power. To be named in the public sphere, apart from some limited instances, was considered appropriate only for the publicity-driven behavior of women who made their living on the stage and were assumed to be immoral, such as the famed dancer Lola Montez. Little had changed since the late eighteenth century, when Georgiana, the Duchess of Devonshire, discovered that a male politician could be a man of the people, but the female equivalent could not shake off the overtones of being a "public woman," a prostitute.[21] Given that her statistics on the Crimean War casualties revealed the importance of sanitation, Nightingale's fame also put her in an impossible position. She was publicly credited a success but was only too aware of the initial disastrous months when so many men had needlessly died. To live in the glare of such an unreal and at least partly false reputation imposed tremendous strain on someone as scrupulous as Nightingale. To take over a nursing school under such conditions and in the spotlight of such unreal expectations was untenable, quite apart from her ill health.

A third factor preventing Nightingale's direct involvement in the proposed training school was that, as she repeatedly insisted, her time was already fully occupied. During 1856–59 she was busy with the Royal Commission into the Army, through which she hoped to achieve much-needed reforms. As it was nearing its close, she initiated a second Royal Commission (1858–63) on the British army in India. Like most of her contemporaries, Nightingale was deeply shocked by the Indian Mutiny of 1857–58. It was the "decisive incentive" for her commitment to reforming the army in India. She then gradually became aware of the plight of Indians under British rule, resulting in an obsession with Indian reform that lasted the rest of her life.[22]

India, the "jewel of the empire," made a huge impact on British sensibilities. India was the home to the exotic, from maharajahs to tigers and elephants. Its fabulous wealth was reflected in the fortunes made by Englishmen ("nabobs") and symbolized by the magnificent Koh-i-noor diamond given to Queen Victoria by the East India Company in 1850. As Nightingale worked alone in her bedroom on such prosaic matters as sanitation, India's exotic allure helped to engage her imagination and emotion. India, for all these reasons, joined with the reform of the army and nursing in providing Nightingale with the wider sense of purpose that she so radically claimed as every woman's right.[23]

The Nightingale Training School for Nurses

Monica Baly outlines how the Nightingale Fund came to found its training school at St. Thomas' Hospital.[24] It was not an obvious choice, as St. Thomas' was neither "well-managed" nor "progressive."[25] Nightingale was won over by her admiration for Sarah Wardroper, the matron, and Richard Whitfield, the resident doctor who, according to Baly, "supplemented his income" by teaching nurses.[26] Accordingly, the Nightingale Fund acceded to St. Thomas' demand that Wardroper be head of the Nightingale Training School as well as continue as matron of the hospital. The combined role proved to be too much for Wardroper, but in Nightingale's opinion, while it was "not the best conceivable way of beginning," it was "the best possible."[27] In 1867, seven years after the school opened, Nightingale's view had not changed. She believed that "our Nurse School is at St. T's simply because Mr. Whitfield & Mrs. Wardroper are there. Every other Officer of the Hospl. is simply a reason for me why it should not be there.... We should take it away but for [them]."[28] Her highly ambivalent feelings about St. Thomas' were reflected in her refusal—with one brief, ceremonial exception in 1881—to make the short journey from her London home to visit it or her school there.

In its early years the most striking aspect of the Nightingale School was its continuity with past practice.[29] The instruction the probationer nurses received was minimal, and there was a high dropout rate. Of the fifteen in the first intake, only four were still nursing a year after completing their training. Results were little better in the following years, but according to Baly, Nightingale "seems not to have noticed."[30]

One reason for Nightingale's lack of observation was, as Baly argues, her preoccupation with the reform of the army. Another reason was her grief over the deaths of close friends and colleagues, including Arthur Clough, first secretary of the Nightingale Fund, and Sir Sidney Herbert, secretary of state at war during the Crimean War (both of whom died in 1861). Yet another reason was that any instruction at all was an improvement for most hospital nurses. Additionally, the Nightingale School encouraged nurses to be conscientious, admitted those who were at least functionally literate, and transferred many of the nurses' traditional cleaning duties to the domestic staff, thus enabling a focus on patient care. Such nurses were desperately needed, especially after the introduction of anesthetics, which allowed more complicated surgery but required demanding postoperative nursing.[31] The result was an ever-increasing demand for nurses with any training at all.

In these vital founding years of the early 1860s, with Nightingale an absentee and preoccupied patron, it was Matron Sarah Wardroper who had the most influence on what we now consider to be "Nightingale nursing." There is little evidence, for example, that Nightingale's systematic approach to teaching nursing skills was implemented in these years.[32] Wardroper and Nightingale were initially in total agreement about another hallmark of "Nightingale nursing": military-style discipline. Such an assumption was evident in other Victorian institutions, including schools and, at times, the family. Thus Nightingale advised that it was "necessary to exact implicit obedience from them [nurses] in little things as well as in great."[33] Nightingale only gradually realized that Wardroper did not balance her discipline with impartial kindness, with what Nightingale called a "motherly" management style.[34] That is a misleading term for modern readers brought up in nuclear, servantless families. Nightingale's experience of mothering was one in which servants provided the hands-on care while mothers were more remote but caring authority figures. Nightingale's concept of mothering was more comparable to the maternal idealization of the fertile but autocratic Queen Victoria, and also quite different from the maternal feminism of the fin de siècle.

By 1868, some eight years after the founding of the Nightingale Training School, Nightingale was forced to realize the extent of its deficiencies and the discrepancies between her vision for nursing and that implemented by Wardroper. In 1866, however, she remained confident that she had safely delegated to Wardroper and Whitfield the task of implementing her concept of nursing while she busied herself with other reforms.

Sydney

In 1866 Henry Parkes, colonial secretary of New South Wales, wrote to Nightingale asking her to send nurses with "an efficient training" to reform Sydney Hospital and be "the Hospital instructors of...female attendants...from which similar charitable institutions in the Country Districts may be supplied."[35] Her first response was cool, as she thought this was yet another demand for nurses that the Nightingale Training School could not supply.

New South Wales, with its relative insignificance and recent past as a penal colony, was far removed from the glamour of India. Yet it still represented escape, and Nightingale, along with many other young women, had dreamed of civilizing such outposts. Most importantly, New South Wales was part of the British Empire. Although Nightingale was aware of the arguments of the many anti-imperialists, her commitment to public service firmly encompassed a responsibility to the empire. Like other reformers, she was spurred on by a vision of an enlightened empire of healthy subjects.[36] The Nightingales were a typical British family of the era in that at least one family member had emigrated, and she had numerous family connections with Australia.[37] In particular, Nightingale's cousin, indispensable adviser, and secretary of the Nightingale Fund from 1861 to 1914 was Henry Bonham Carter; his wife, Sibella, regularly corresponded with her "great friend" and cousin Elizabeth Onslow, the daughter of a prominent colonial family who lived outside Sydney.[38]

When considering Parkes's request, Nightingale drew not just on her wealth of family-related experiences but also on her own. During 1863–65 she had been particularly involved in Australian concerns. She had supported Lady (Harriet) Dowling, the wife of a chief justice of New South Wales, in her efforts to encourage British nurses to emigrate to

Australia and New Zealand.[39] Nightingale had included Australia in her concern for the plight of the empire's indigenous populations and in 1864 published her "Note on the Aboriginal Races of Australia."[40] In 1865, at the request of the English social reformer Maria Rye, Nightingale had lobbied to reform conditions at the Gladesville Asylum, Sydney's main psychiatric institution.[41]

Nightingale therefore entered negotiations with Parkes unusually well informed. She also believed she owed Australians a debt of gratitude. Throughout the nineteenth century Australian colonists were consistently generous donors to appeals from Britain, and they had reacted with typical generosity (or determination to prove their worth) to the Nightingale Fund appeal. A decade later Nightingale showed she had been sincere when responding to the donations to the fund made by the colonists in South Australia: "England is one wherever her people dwell. That your hearts were with us in our struggles & will be with us always, we know with a gratitude which will not pass away."[42]

The request from Parkes also came when Nightingale was despairing of implementing nursing reform in India. The year before, she had carefully drawn up a scheme to train nurses under the auspices of the Indian government. In 1867, after two years' delay by the authorities, came the confirmation that her painstakingly designed scheme had been enlarged and then rejected as impractical. It was a "bitter blow" to Nightingale's dream of extending nursing reform to India.[43] With the approach from the New South Wales government, Nightingale had another chance to disseminate nursing reform from, she still believed, its successful base at St. Thomas' Hospital.

Nightingale's hopes were soon bolstered by the flattering deference shown to her by Parkes and other Australian officials. Another major factor was Parkes's open-handed munificence—almost indifference—regarding the cost of the scheme. Nightingale also responded favorably to the main medical promoter of the scheme, the surgeon Alfred Roberts. Roberts had drawn up the memorandum that Parkes had attached to his original letter to Nightingale, summarizing the request and giving basic information about Sydney Hospital. Nightingale deeply appreciated logical thinking and precise information, as in Roberts's memo. It was Wardroper who pointed out the "missing link" in the scheme suggested by Roberts: he proposed to have ward sisters who would be supervised by the hospital surgeon, as practiced by his alma mater, Guy's Hospital in London. On Wardroper's urging, Nightingale insisted that a matron be appointed who would supervise the nurses: for Nightingale, this became the most important plank in "Nightingale nursing."[44]

After prolonged negotiations the Nightingale Fund authorized six nurses to go to Sydney. It was a remarkable sign of Nightingale's commitment, as only 102 nurses had completed their training by the end of 1866, so the six comprised almost 6 percent of the school's total output. It was also more like 12 percent of available nurses since, according to Baly, only around fifty Nightingale nurses still nursed in hospitals a decade after the school was founded.[45]

Wardroper chose Lucy Osburn to head the team of nurses when Osburn was just a month into her year-long training. The choice was made on the basis of Osburn's status as a "lady" and her supposed nursing experience. Osburn wanted such a post because, as Wardroper told Nightingale, she "cannot live in our ever varying climate and on the score of health will be glad to leave England."[46] Despite some four months' absence due to illness, she formally completed her training on 29 September 1867. A little over two months later she sailed for Sydney with five other Nightingale nurses. Osburn set out with all the assumptions of a naive imperialist: that she, as an English lady, was far superior to the colonials and so could reform their nursing and take over the management of Sydney Hospital. Yet she soon had her assumptions shaken as she encountered capable matrons and met people far from the rough, ignorant figures of her imagination. In particular, Henry Parkes became an avuncular mentor.[47]

Osburn was soon aware how sadly ill-prepared she was for her task of reforming colonial nursing.[48] The unrealistic expectations of her as the Lady of the Lamp's representative were further inflated by her role in helping to nurse Prince Alfred, Queen Victoria's second son, when he was shot by a would-be assassin a week after Osburn arrived in Sydney.[49] Osburn reacted by clinging to two bedrocks in her sea of uncertainty. One was her assumption that Nightingale would be impressed by Osburn's easy acceptance by the colonial elite. The second was that there was little difference between Nightingale's concept of nursing and that practiced by the Sisters of St. John's House. Osburn was seriously wrong on both counts.

Florence Nightingale and Lucy Osburn had met a few times but only after Osburn had completed her training and was preparing to leave for Australia. For Nightingale, her family's social standing and her own fame meant that she could take her status for granted. She was, after all, someone whom even royalty, including the Crown Princess of Prussia,

Queen Victoria's eldest and much admired daughter, clamored to visit and meekly accepted the conditions she imposed.[50] In contrast, Osburn's childhood had been marked by economic insecurity, which meant she could never take her social position for granted. She was deeply impressed by her acceptance by Sydney society, and a major theme of her letters to Nightingale was her friendships with the elite women of Sydney. Osburn remained oblivious that Nightingale was completely indifferent to this aspect of Osburn's life. Nor did Nightingale consider that any imprimatur other than her own was needed for her nursing reforms. Few of Nightingale's letters to Osburn have survived, but Nightingale was consistent in encouraging details and precise plans while appreciating requests for advice. Disastrously, Osburn's letters only incidentally mentioned such matters.

Osburn's second assumption—that there was little difference between Nightingale's concept of nursing and that of the Sisters of St. John's House—was an understandable mistake. Osburn, like many other Nightingale nurses, had gained midwifery experience under the Sisters of St. John at King's College Hospital after completing her training at St. Thomas'. Mary Jones, the lady superior of the sisters, was a major influence on Nightingale's concept of nursing. Yet there was one key difference: any nursing promoted by the Nightingale Fund had to be nonsectarian. Nightingale understood this thoroughly, with all the instincts and knowledge of a born and seasoned politician and, since the Crimean War, an experienced administrator. The comparatively sheltered Osburn arrived in Sydney with little realization that as an employee of the colonial government, she needed to be demonstratively nonsectarian. Nor did she understand the determination of the colonists to found secular, rather than church-run, public institutions. Osburn's High Church beliefs offended the most powerful group on the Board of Sydney Hospital, the Evangelicals. Osburn had been rebelling against her family's Evangelicalism since her teens. She initially had no recognition that what she had done in England as a private person was very different from her behavior in Sydney as a public employee and Nightingale's representative. A series of disastrous actions inflamed Evangelical hostility toward Osburn, culminating in her order to a groundsman at Sydney Hospital to burn some old bibles—seen as the ultimate anti-Protestant act. Some five months away by return of mail, Nightingale could only watch helplessly as her cherished concept of a nursing service motivated by Christianity yet above sectarianism was undermined in Sydney by Osburn.[51]

These were just two of the initial problems Nightingale had with Osburn, but initially Nightingale clung to one great consolation: Osburn's
intense admiration for Wardroper and the Nightingale Training School.
Effectively motherless from a young age, Osburn saw Wardroper as
her "dear Mother at St. Thomas."[52] As Nightingale confided to Bonham
Carter, Osburn "was never weary of speaking...with affectionate pride,
of 'my training' 'our training at St. Thomas.'" Furthermore, Osburn reassured Nightingale by maintaining that the nurses at St. Thomas' were the
only nurses to get "real training" and that "the amount & kind of knowledge given at St. Thomas' to the Nurses was exactly...right."[53]

Yet the chorus of complaint about Wardroper's management increased.
Nightingale earnestly believed that nurses needed character training as
much as clinical skills, an assumption that came to characterize British
nursing education.[54] Yet by 1867 she doubted that her Training School
provided any character training at all. She was outraged when the Swed-
ish Emmy Rappe, who trained with Osburn, was reported as saying that
the school would teach an experienced nurse only to be more "obedient
and humble" but no new nursing skills. Nightingale believed the opposite: that the school taught nursing skills but it was "quite doubtful" that
it improved the nurses' characters. Nightingale added, "I never let even
my left hand hear me think so."[55] It was a jocular remark but one that
accurately pointed to her determined effort to shut her mind against the
growing evidence that things were seriously wrong.

Soon Nightingale was faced with more complaints. She could no longer hide from the appalling possibility that the school, with which she
was so publicly and irretrievably associated, did little to teach clinical
skills *or* improve character. Would it be the Crimean War all over again,
where she achieved public adulation for efforts that, in her own mind,
were a tragic failure?

In mid-1868 Maria Dimsdale and three other unnamed nurses accused
Wardroper of unkind treatment, arbitrary conduct, and a lack of any
systematic training. As Dimsdale had also trained with Osburn, Night-
ingale wrote asking for her opinion. Nightingale was reassured when
Osburn warmly rejected Dimsdale as being too self-interested for a good
Nightingale nurse.[56] Nightingale was not only again lulled but buoyed
by a similar comment from one of her most trusted advisers, Dr. John
Sutherland, one of the members of the Sanitary Commission during the
Crimean War. Sutherland suggested that the issue was not Wardroper's
management but rather that of "self willed women" who lacked a sense

of "vocation." He advised Nightingale that they should teach the concept of vocation to all nurses at the school.[57] Thus Wardroper's erratic management helped to make the concept of a nursing "vocation" a keystone of Nightingale nursing. Difficulties were now seen as tests of vocation, and criticisms were again dismissed.

Yet still the accusations kept coming. Nightingale shut herself away from her adoring public but, like many Victorian women, had intense friendships. From girlhood, particular women had been idolized friends until, inevitably, they failed to live up to her expectations. One of her nurses whom she most admired in the mid-1860s was Elizabeth Torrance. When Torrance supported the complaints about Wardroper and the lack of instruction at the Nightingale Training School, Nightingale could no longer ignore the problem. Then she discovered that her other mainstay of the school, Richard Whitfield, who was meant to lecture the probationers, was neglectful and "untrustworthy."[58] Nightingale had previously judged Osburn as the "the only one we trained...who was a woman of purpose & courage."[59] Now it was Osburn's "very ordinary" character that had caused her to sink to the level of the most inferior nurse at St. Thomas'; Osburn's appointment to Sydney was just one of the "the inevitable mistakes" arising from Wardroper's poor judgment.[60]

When Nightingale eventually faced the problem of the Nightingale School, she did so squarely, recording her deep distress at Wardroper's mental state, the probationers' overwork and poor conditions, and the unpleasant tone in the Nurses' Home.[61] Nightingale was outraged to discover that Wardroper taught the nurses to stop any patient care and stand at attention when she entered a ward. As Nightingale wrote to Bonham Carter, she would have no more thought of demanding that at Scutari than asking a surgeon to stop an operation if she entered the room.[62]

Nightingale had no power to dismiss Wardroper, and both her warm humanity and pragmatism prompted her to respond to Wardroper's tearful appeals for support. Nightingale forgave and continued to work with Wardroper, but Osburn was a different matter. Nightingale moved in circles where those who transgressed the strict social codes were routinely ostracized.[63] Osburn could defend herself only by letter, and did so clumsily as she did not realize that Nightingale had so dramatically revised her opinion of Wardroper. As late as 1873, Osburn wrote imploringly to Nightingale, assuring her, "If Mrs. Wardroper was popped down in our Hospital tomorrow morn[in]g. except for the local differences & smaller number she w[oul]d not know it from her own."[64] She had no idea that that was just what Nightingale feared. Osburn made matters worse when she reported her success in training colonial nurses while condemning as inadequate the five other Nightingale School–trained nurses who had accompanied her to Australia. Nightingale was disillusioned with Wardroper but still could not tolerate the implication that even a nurse as inadequate as Osburn could produce better nurses than her own school. That the Nightingale School recruited British women while Osburn trained (mere) colonials added to the insult.[65]

The combined result was that Nightingale showed her harshest side to Osburn. She effectively cut Osburn adrift—neither the first nor the last time she reacted in this way. Nightingale had Bonham Carter write to Osburn that she would no longer reply to any of her letters. Osburn was devastated, but there is no indication that Nightingale relented during the eleven more years Osburn spent in Sydney. Nightingale also tried to expunge Osburn's very real achievements as the founder of trained nursing for Australian women from the Nightingale Fund's reports. Further, she consistently referred to Osburn as the worst possible nurse, even in comparison with those she considered troublemaking drug addicts. Australia, once a land of promise, was similarly condemned. No nurse was worse than Lucy Osburn, and few places worse than Sydney.[66]

The savagery of Nightingale's reactions was personal but also a response to the potential for Osburn to demonstrate the failings of the Nightingale School. It can additionally be accounted for by the deep blow that Osburn, along with the Indian government, dealt to her dream of reforming nursing throughout the empire. The Sydney project had gone from a model to be emulated to a disaster to forget. Osburn's admiration of Wardroper was now merely a symptom of underlying problems—ones that, at St. Thomas', could not be so easily dismissed. Once they were acknowledged, frantic efforts were made to rectify them. In 1872 Whitfield was replaced, steps were taken for probationers finally to be given systematic instruction, and Nightingale began her famous annual addresses exhorting the probationers to higher ideals. The next year Nightingale arranged for the probationers to visit her in order to form her own judgment and to influence them.

The biggest issue remained Wardroper's deleterious influence on the nurses. A compromise solution was found with the appointment of a "Home Sister" to care for and educate the probationers.[67] The first home sister was the admired Nightingale nurse who had helped convince Nightingale of the problem: Elizabeth Torrance. Torrance took up the position in 1872 but, much to Nightingale's disappointment, left within months to get married. Torrance's successor also did not last long.[68] Again, Nightingale faced a repetition of her Crimean War nightmare of public triumph and private disaster. Exposure of the problems of the Nightingale Training School also risked the destruction of Nightingale's influence and hence other reform projects. Then Nightingale found another ideal home sister: Maria Machin.

Canada

Nightingale's propensity to idolize selected friends found another outlet in Maria Machin, a widely traveled Canadian and experienced teacher cum school principal.[69] Machin entered the Nightingale Training School on 25 March 1873 highly recommended by one of the most eminent women in Nightingale's circle of friends: Frances, Baroness de Bunsen, whose husband had been the Prussian ambassador to the English Court of St. James.[70] Nightingale had the "most affectionate & reverential love" for Bunsen, and her admiration soon encompassed Machin. When Bunsen died in 1876, Nightingale told Machin that her friend's great contribution had been that "she gave us you."[71] In a further contrast to Osburn, a month after she began her training Machin not only recognized but was confident enough to write to Nightingale about the problems within the school.[72] In a note on Machin's entry in the Probationers' Record Book, Nightingale endorsed Machin as embodying her ideal nurse: "the highest character & most spiritual tone & purpose, excepting Agnes Jones, that we have had in this work:—Chastened in spirit: of masculine determination & education: experienced in life & its trials:—unflinching in resolution to carry out God's work:—we have never had anyone so fitted to exercise the highest influence over women."[73]

By August 1873, five months after Machin had begun her training, Nightingale wrote addressing her as "my dear friend" and closing with "God bless you, my dear friend....Ever yours overflowingly, Florence Nightingale." Such effusion of emotion was within the friendship norm for Nightingale. It helped to bind both men and women to her in loving and supportive servitude; the most productive of these relationships was the one with Sir Sidney Herbert, the secretary of state at war during the Crimean War, and the secretary of the Nightingale Fund, Henry Bonham Carter. Nightingale's female friends were equally important, and conventions allowed much more explicit declarations of love between platonic female friends than now.[74] Her expressions of love for Machin add little to our knowledge of Nightingale's sexuality. Our category of "lesbian" is notoriously difficult to apply to past ages with their very different consciousness of female sexuality. In the case of the relationships between Nightingale and her female friends, the balance of probability is that it was another example of intense friendship between women who self-identified either as heterosexual or as natural celibates. It is relevant also that Nightingale did not view such friendships exclusively. She habitually referred to Elizabeth Vincent, an intimate friend of Machin's and also a Nightingale-trained nurse, as "David," thereby comparing Vincent's and Machin's friendship with the biblical one of David and Jonathan. Whatever the underlying sexuality, the female relationships were understood to be passionately intense. Nightingale accepted without question, for instance, Vincent's assumption that an illness of Nightingale's had been caused by worry over Machin's health.[75]

It was in her letter of August 1873 that Nightingale implored Machin to take the position of home sister. "With regard to the 'Home' duty...I am almost afraid to write about it...I dare hardly hope. It seems almost too good to be true." Nightingale argued that personal attachment would solve any difficulties since, although Wardroper might resent Machin's appointment, "in her heart" she would be glad because "she is very fond of you." Character training, Nightingale told Machin, was desperately needed "in that poor [Nurses'] 'Home'": "I have seen women—& quite as much Nurses as Ladies,—come into our 'Home' with the highest aspirations & religious motives—And, because they did not find...the supporting & raising influence in this 'Home'—they fell off. And because they did not find the good they sought, thought there was no good." Nightingale was confident that Machin was the kind of "woman who can 'mother' & train other women." She ended with the flattery that she so effectively used to cajole others to work for her causes: Nightingale noted how, as Machin's health improved, she "looked so beautiful" and how her own "anxiety changed into admiration."[76]

It is indicative of Nightingale's priorities that she did not mention Machin's glaring deficiency: she was even less experienced as a nurse than Osburn. Within weeks of beginning her training, Machin had developed an infected finger, which meant that "her attendance in the Ward was too irregular to permit any report from the Sister." She returned to work, but her probationer's record indicates that she again became ill and was absent from July to November. On 5 November she returned to St. Thomas' "but in consequence of previous severe illness was not allowed to resume her ward training."[77] The result was that Machin had just two months' instruction, more than most nurses but much less than the year's training expected of a Nightingale nurse.

Much to Nightingale's delight, Machin accepted the position of home sister, beginning on Christmas Day 1873. As Nightingale had shown her implacable side to Osburn, she now revealed her capacity for intense gratitude. For Nightingale, fourteen years after the Nightingale Training School had been founded, Machin's appointment marked its effective beginning: a school that now improved character as well as taught nursing. Nightingale privately assured Machin that she had "set us up in the Home at St. Thomas'. We always look upon you as its creator."[78] Nightingale was also effusive in her public praise. In her address to her probationer nurses in 1875, she praised Machin for having made the Nurses' Home "a place of real training of character, habits, intelligence...a place something like what a 'Training Home' ought to be," where Machin provided the probationers with "mothering care."[79]

Nightingale's capacity for generosity was tested in 1875 when Machin decided to return to Canada. Montreal General Hospital had agreed to the urging of its medical staff and requested a team of St. Thomas'–trained nurses to reform nursing and train other nurses. It was much the same scenario as Sydney but with an important difference: it was not a government-funded project, and Nightingale did not see it as the beginning of an officially sponsored dissemination of reformed nursing throughout the empire. Rather, she viewed it as a personal favor to Machin for her saving of the Training School.

Nightingale initially insisted that the Nightingale Fund would not allow any of their nurses to go with Machin to Montreal until they had received a firm commitment that the hospital would be rebuilt. She made this clear to Machin: "I do most solemnly say: don't commit yourself to Montreal on any such [vague] understanding...I do most emphatically say that...I consider it our duty to decline letting them have our Nurses till we see what improvements in accommodation and construction they propose to make in black & white...I think it simply impossible to let Nurses go to that Montreal Hospital til we know what they will do to improve it."[80] Extensive improvements were made to the hospital. During 1873–77, Can$43,000 was spent to transform the "old and decrepit building into a reasonably modern institution." Even then, Montreal

General was still far less than Nightingale's dream of a "model hospital" for Machin.[81]

Machin and four Nightingale nurses began work at Montreal General Hospital on 2 October 1875. By then Osburn was halfway through her time in Sydney and would spend another seven years trying to implement Nightingale nursing and training nurses while cut off from Nightingale's support. Machin had gone to Montreal despite Nightingale's misgivings, but Nightingale remained warmly supportive. One letter by Nightingale to Machin began, "If I were to write to you as often as I think of you, I should always be writing." She told Machin how "so very anxious" she was about her but how she had been relieved to hear that at Montreal General Hospital, Machin's "word is Law...as it ought to be." She affirmed her faith in Machin's future career: "I have the greatest faith in your 'star.'"[82] Despite setbacks, Nightingale remained positive. She assured Machin that generally "yours is a success & that you are doing so much good," and, "Your troubles are continually before me but also your successes."[83]

In 1877 Nightingale helped to select two more nurses from St. Thomas' to join Machin at Montreal. Soon after, a committee of the Montreal General Hospital recommended that Machin's three-year contract as lady superintendent not be renewed. The decision was made on financial grounds during an economic depression and was partly justified by Machin's failure to begin a training school for nurses.[84] Machin's improvements in the standard of the nursing had, however, resulted in the support of the Medical Board, which helped to reverse the decision.[85] Nevertheless, Machin was bruised by such public controversy, and the failure of the hospital to publicly defend her against charges in an anonymous pamphlet was the last straw. Machin and the remaining Nightingale nurses resigned, leaving on 30 June 1878. So the first systematic attempt to spread Nightingale nursing to Canada ended within three years. As Machin had not trained nurses, she had little lasting impact on Canadian nursing.[86]

As coldly hostile as Nightingale had been to Osburn in her troubles, she was warm and loving to Machin. The comparison was stark. In 1874 Nightingale wrote to Henry Bonham Carter about the danger of nurses reading medical texts, illustrating it with the example of Osburn, who had used them to give "Lectures at Sydney!!! on anatomy!"[87] Yet five months later Nightingale presented Machin with the two-volume work *The Practice of Medicine,* inscribing on it: "Offered to our dear Miss Machin by (I would say: by her warmest admirer but she would not let me) by one who offers up daily thanks to the Almighty Father for having called her to the Training of women to help Christ in the care of the sick."[88]

The comparison of Nightingale's attitude toward Osburn, by now quietly successful in Sydney, with Machin was also explicit: "You cannot think with what gratitude to our Father I acknowledge the different feelings with which I think of our Nurses going to you: & [compared with] to some of our Matrons to whom we used to send nurses in the Colonies & elsewhere." She added, "Of those Thou hast given me I have not lost one! I know you will be able to say."[89] Even when Machin did "lose" some of her Nightingale-trained nurses by dismissing them, it made no difference to Nightingale's warmth.

Nightingale's letters to Machin, despite their conventional formality in forms of address ("Miss Machin" and "Miss Nightingale"), show the extent to which she idolized Machin. Nightingale's devotion made her a warm, generous, and tactful friend and mentor. When Machin faced dismissal and failure, Nightingale did not lessen her support, writing, "Dearest friend Miss Machin, 'Let not your heart be troubled': was not Christ's life on earth to all human appearance on the day of his death a failure? And shall we have any right to say that ours is?" Nightingale advised Machin not to make a hasty decision to resign, but she would not countenance the St. Thomas'–trained nurses staying on without Machin's supervision. So firm was she on this point that she offered to pay the cost of their trip back to England herself if the Nightingale Fund would not. Nightingale also consoled Machin on the death of her supporter and "young friend," the house surgeon Dr. Cline, ending her letter, "If love were heavy, I must charter a A1 steamer with love to yourself: ever yours in God's name F Nightingale."[90]

As the crisis at Montreal deepened, Nightingale's support for Machin remained firm. She drew on their shared Christian faith for consolation: "It is terrible for me this Montreal disaster & what you are going thro'. But never mind: the Lord will bear it for us.... Now kiss me across the Atlantic: God holds our hands together."[91] Finally, she supported Machin's decision to leave "a place connected with so much suffering & injustice to you," trusting Machin's judgment: "So truly I am sure that you & God are the only judges." While Nightingale condemned Osburn's bad management as creating delinquent nurses, she assured Machin that "worthy" nurses on her staff would remain loyal: if they did not, they were, ipso facto, unworthy.[92] The last letter Nightingale sent before Machin resigned modeled her belief in motherly concern for the individual: "Dearest, I am only afraid of events being too much for your health. Pray try to preserve it. I feel as if I had not told you enough how much your trials are mine. It is not far away but near, very near, in my heart that I feel your trials.... Dearest, we meet in God's heart: & in this heart I leave you. To Him I commit myself & you who are far dearer."[93]

Nightingale's generous, loving friendship continued after Machin returned to London. She started to again refer to her friend as "Home Sister," which tactfully reminded Machin of her success in that post rather than her failure in Montreal.[94] Nightingale also showed her tact in dealing with Machin's comparative poverty: "Dearest, if expense is a difficulty let me have the pleasure—you know we are such old friends—... of paying your fare back here for a flying visit."[95] Even more practically, she supported Machin's appointment as matron of the prestigious London hospital St. Bartholomew's. In contrast, when Lucy Osburn finally returned to London after seventeen years in Sydney, Nightingale relented sufficiently to allow her to visit but there is no indication that she gave Osburn any other assistance.

Conclusion

Nightingale had far from an easy path in reforming nursing. The responsibility for the Nightingale Training School was, as she pointed out, thrust upon her. Her frequent complaints of being overworked could be manipulative and sound bizarrely egotistical when directed to Henry Bonham Carter, who had a career, a large family, and the burden of managing the Nightingale Fund. Yet it was nevertheless true. Busy with army reform, India, and countless demands for her assistance, Nightingale tried her best to ignore the deficiencies of her school. Eventually, the criticisms became too numerous and too credible.

Lucy Osburn's difficulties in Sydney helped to prick the bubble of complacency with which Nightingale viewed her school. When Nightingale finally realized the full extent of its problems, she was devastated, and Osburn's wholehearted admiration for it and for Matron Wardroper only made the situation worse. There were good reasons for Nightingale's despair. Her unprecedented celebrity and the public donations that had supported the Nightingale Fund meant that if the Nightingale Training School failed, it would do so in the fullest glare of publicity. That it appeared a public triumph while concealing severe problems also had uncomfortable echoes with Nightingale's initial months at Scutari Hospital. As well, these revelations and Osburn's misjudgments in Sydney combined to shatter any hope Nightingale had of the school being an effective base from which to disseminate her style of reformed nursing throughout the empire. The result was that the early 1870s disintegrated into a nightmare for Nightingale.

Maria Machin appeared as the savior who rescued Nightingale from public ignominy. As the home sister, she transformed the Nightingale School and its nurse probationers. Machin was much more overt in her spirituality than Osburn, and Nightingale idolized her as an ideal nurse who cared for the sick from a divine vocation. When Machin went to Canada, Nightingale's support was the gesture of a loving mentor. Accordingly, when Machin resigned, Nightingale viewed it as a private disappointment, not as another blow to her hopes to nurse the empire. Additionally, from the mid-1870s Nightingale's health slowly improved and she began to see more visitors. For all these reasons, Machin brought out the very best in Nightingale, who consistently acted as her warm, loving, patient friend and generous mentor.

The intensity of Nightingale's response to Osburn and Machin was heightened by her situation as a deeply passionate and visionary genius who was also an invalid. She felt herself to be, in her words, "a prisoner" to her bed and illness. Her passion for empire and friendship provided an intellectual and emotional outlet that transcended her bedroom (and gender). Yet the limitations of the Nightingale School under Wardroper distorted Nightingale's contribution to nursing reform. It also blighted her dream of using the Nightingale Fund to send teams of nurses to disseminate nursing reform throughout the empire. The two attempts to do so, in Australia and Canada, reflect the bedridden Nightingale's intense but flawed reliance on selected individuals to ensure the success of her vision for reforming nursing. When reformed nursing swept the world, it would do so in Nightingale's name, but in a far more haphazard way than she initially dreamed.

RHETORIC AND REALITY IN AMERICA

JOAN E. LYNAUGH

Ask anyone in the United States to name a famous nurse, and he or she will respond, "I can think of only one—Florence Nightingale." Nightingale's iconic status does indeed prevail in the United States, where "Nurses Week" is celebrated around May 12 to memorialize Nightingale's 1820 birth date. If we turn to an Internet search for word on Nightingale, we get about 1,300,000 hits. Should we take this fame to mean that nursing in the United States descends from Nightingale's ideas and influence? I explore that question by examining the origins and chronology of nineteenth- and early twentieth-century modern "trained" nursing in the United States.

Emergence of the Trained Nurse

The evolution of modern nursing in the United States now spans about 170 years. Early in the nineteenth century some people, most of whom were women, began to offer their services as nurses by advertising to their communities in trade directories. The illnesses, injuries, and displacements associated with urban life and industrial work created demand for reliable caretakers. On the other side of the equation were women seeking respectable and gainful employment. Nursing was an everyday part of domestic life, so it is not surprising that some women would be attracted to the idea of earning a living by caring for others. As historian Susan Reverby points out, a "professed nurse" often began by nursing her family, then developed proficiency and obtained work by word of mouth.[1]

Fairly soon, however, reformers began to see that reliance on family caregiving and this informal system of professed caretakers left many citizens vulnerable or even abandoned to their fate. Factory and commercial employment, which separated home from work, limited the ability of the family to cope without serious financial loss. Migrants from rural areas or foreign countries often did not even have the option of extended family support. Well before the Civil War new approaches, from reformers both religious and secular, began to surface regarding care of the sick in their own homes or in institutions.

In 1839, for instance, Dr. Joseph Warrington, a Quaker, organized the Philadelphia Nurse Society to send nurses into the home to care for women during and after childbirth. Warrington wanted to upgrade the quality of care for poor women and to make this form of nursing work respectable and reliable. Later, in 1861, Ann Preston, another Quaker physician, opened a training school for nurses at Woman's Hospital in Philadelphia. Preston outlined her ideas of what nurses needed to know in her 1863 book *Nursing the Sick and the Training of Nurses*.[2] Progress on the school was interrupted by the demands of the Civil War. Returning from her volunteer work nursing soldiers, the first American-trained nurse, Harriet Newton Phillips, received her diploma from Woman's Hospital after six months of study in 1869.

Nursing by women members of religious orders spread across the country in the nineteenth century. The Sisters of Charity, the Sisters of Mercy, the Lutheran Deaconesses, the Sisters of St. Joseph, and several other orders of nursing sisters opened hospitals or nursed the sick in their homes in various American cities before 1850. Most of these groups originated in Ireland, Germany, or France and emigrated or were recruited to the United States along with the thousands of European immigrants flooding into the country. The religious women found women to join their ranks among these immigrants and soon became a significant factor in the spread of hospitals and nursing. Their patterns of care and the design of their hospitals reflected the institutions and mores of their native lands, but they adapted successfully to the economic and political practices of the United States.[3]

The Hospital Idea

Hospitals proliferated in every American community after the mid-nineteenth century. Almost all these new institutions were private, non-governmental enterprises, often built on ethnic or religious foundations. As the hospital idea spread, many towns and small cities supported more than one hospital. For instance, there might be a small hospital funded by the local Lutherans or Presbyterians or Episcopalians. A few blocks away, the local Roman Catholics, perhaps of Irish or German descent, opened their own hospital. Patients were expected to pay for care if they could, but the day-to-day costs of running the hospital and paying caretakers fell on voluntary hospital supporters. At first, these hospitals were housed in converted homes; later, large edifices symbolic of civic virtue were built for the successful ones.

In larger cities there were public hospitals, of course, which usually depended on city or county taxes or sometimes state subsidies. These public hospitals were intended to care for the poor, the insane, and the deviants of the city and often began as almshouses. Several, such as Bellevue in New York City, Charity Hospital in New Orleans, and Philadelphia Hospital in Philadelphia, endured vociferous public criticism as they struggled with the serious problem of finding caretakers for their ever-growing numbers of patients.

A Link with Nightingale

One of these struggling hospitals, the Philadelphia Hospital, provides a significant link with Florence Nightingale which may help us consider Nightingale's impact on American nursing. Alice Fisher, an 1876 graduate of St. Thomas' School in London, was sought out by Philadelphia's Guardians of the Poor, who were charged with responsibility for the management of the three-thousand-bed city hospital. In the mid-1880s the hospital was racked by scandals, deeply embarrassing the Guardians, who included many of Philadelphia's leading citizens. The food was bad, graft and stealing were common, and the patients were disorderly, even to the point of committing murder. To stem the crisis, the Guardians launched a search to find a superintendent able to create order among these most destitute of people. They consulted Henry Bonham Carter, secretary of the Nightingale Fund, who, it was said, suggested Alice Fisher, an experienced graduate of the St. Thomas' School. Fisher arrived in 1885 with an impressive record of prior successes in workhouse reform.

Fisher's reform strategies relied on close collaboration with her advocates among the Guardians, support from local prominent physicians, insistence on trained assistants whom she alone selected, and the immediate creation of a nurses' training school. She was said to have a strong and attractive personality. Her magnetism, confidence, and moral persuasiveness made her very popular with Philadelphia's citizens and newspapers to the extent that she transformed their picture of the hospital from a scandal to a popular cause. Moreover, she was able to build enduring loyalty among her nurses and physician colleagues.

Alice Fisher, who had a history of mitral stenosis, died of what was probably congestive heart failure in 1889. In the brief time she lived in Philadelphia, she built an image and a structure for nursing that lasted for generations. Like Nightingale, she became something of an icon for her successors. She was widely eulogized in the newspapers; memorialized in a large oil painting by Alice Barber, a student of Thomas Eakins; and for fifty years after her death nurses at the Philadelphia Hospital made annual Easter pilgrimages to her grave. In the accounts of the time it seems that for Philadelphians, Fisher represented the morally inspired, intelligent, and committed woman reformer who could help make urban life workable and acceptable.[4]

It is unclear whether Fisher's impact on Philadelphia helps us judge Nightingale's impact on American nursing. It is true that Fisher found her nursing career at St. Thomas', benefited from the Nightingale Fund, and was helped by Nightingale to obtain her first posts after completing her training. And perhaps Nightingale helped Fisher get the post in Philadelphia through Henry Bonham Carter. Fisher's record at St. Thomas' as a lady probationer was good, but her subsequent correspondence with Nightingale is dutiful and polite. And Nightingale's written and verbal references to Fisher range from lukewarm to downright cranky; for example, in one exchange, she complains that Fisher is "a gentlewoman and a literary lady...who knows nothing of nursing."[5] It seems that Fisher's successful career emanated from her opportunity at St. Thomas' Hospital but did not depend on a warm relationship with Nightingale.

Not the Nightingale Model

Moreover, the situation in Philadelphia did not correspond with the Nightingale idea that the nurse leader should be given entire control of the nursing staff, the teaching, and the discipline. In Philadelphia,

Fisher had to contend with and report to not only the Guardians but also the residents and the chief physician of the House Staff. Her budget came from the city, meaning that she had to negotiate all matters of space, the training school, and authority. Her success stemmed from finding an American way to create a new field of work and reform an old institution, using her education, experience, and personal skills.

In the United States, then, the evolution of trained nursing took place in a complex and changing context. The growth of cities and flow of population from rural to urban areas as well as growing demands for sanitary reforms and therapeutic instead of merely palliative care in hospitals drove change in both the mission of hospitals and their importance to the public. The devastating experiences of the Civil War and the significant role of volunteer and paid nurses created a new public image of what could be possible to gain from nursing. After the war, in the 1870s, the rapid spread of training schools was inseparable from the idea of a safe, antiseptically clean, and increasingly therapeutic hospital where surgery was performed, medications administered, and order maintained.

Authority systems in the new training schools, however, as noted above, were different from those of the Nightingale model. The training schools almost never enjoyed independent funding. Most hospitals were governed by volunteer boards of trustees who held authority over medical and nursing personnel. The hospital relied on the relatively inexpensive labor of the pupils in the training school, and the nursing leader was dependent on the administrative and financial stability of the institution. The pupils learned as they worked and usually completed their program in two years, later extended to three years. The nurse superintendent was responsible for the care of the patients and the education and oversight of the pupils. In many nineteenth-century hospitals only one or two graduate nurses supervised and taught the pupils and oversaw patient care.

Except in tax-supported city, county, or state public hospitals, financial stability was a never-ending problem. The boards that managed the private, voluntary majority of hospitals sought to meet their charitable and moral goals of caring for the sick. Many hospitals failed when they found it too hard to manage their deficits by soliciting gifts and voluntary group contributions and by relying on low-cost labor such as that of the pupil nurses. Successful hospitals tried hard to attract paying patients by improving their surgical facilities, offering maternity services, and reaching out to popular physicians so that they might admit their patients. But although these community hospitals were the most common type in the United States, they were, until the twentieth-century advent of hospital insurance, always vulnerable to failure.

Nightingale's Influence

In view of the difficulties of the hospitals, we can wonder how nursing, so dependent on hospitals, managed to grow and more or less prosper through the nineteenth century and into the twentieth. It may be here that the iconic reform message of Nightingale and the power of her ideas played an important, if hard to measure, role. Nightingale's *Notes on Nursing*, first published in the United States in 1860,[6] was required reading for hospital reformers and supporters of the nursing idea. Her name was always attached to accounts of the importance and success of this "new profession for women in America." One classic example of these stories is a twelve-page article in the *Century Magazine* by Franklin D. North. It appeared in November 1882, accompanied by a full-page image of Nightingale and many drawings of nurses at work and patients being carefully attended. North told the middle- and upper-class readers of the magazine that the nurses' training school at Bellevue Hospital, established in 1873 in New York City, was conceived under the direct guidance of Nightingale, a distinctly upper-class Englishwoman. Her message, according to North, was that nursing required an educated, responsible, committed woman willing and able to substitute for the family in its responsibility for the care of the sick. And New Yorkers could trust that all Bellevue nurses met those criteria because the leadership at Bellevue had taken its cue on how to create the school from the heroic, famous, and absolutely credible Florence Nightingale.

The American System

Twenty years after the 1861 opening of the Woman's Hospital Training School for Nurses in Philadelphia, the growing acceptance of hospital-based allopathic medicine served to weld nurses, hospitals, and physicians in a hierarchical embrace. The new nurses and their schools were often sponsored and overseen by elite women or local businessmen. In general, these affluent local leaders viewed the nurses as their agents for social reform, philanthropy, community uplift, and modern health care. And importantly, nursing was seen by many Americans as a promising avenue toward improving the condition of women through respectable work.

Molding young women into reliable nurses, as we have seen, helped solve the care problems of the new hospitals opening in communities across the county. But the training schools yielded another change. As pupil nurses copied their physician lectures into their notebooks, they were able to learn something new and fascinating. Their notebooks became their textbooks. In a way, nineteenth-century physicians' already tentative monopoly on medical knowledge was undermined by this necessary sharing with nurses. Mary Clymer, a graduate of the Training School of the Hospital of the University of Pennsylvania in 1889, saved her notebooks. Evidently she decided to record, on a daily basis, everything she did on the wards, in addition to making careful notes of formal lectures. She reported on her newfound ability to change a bed with a patient in it, she learned about the indications of dropsy, she tried to keep a typhoid patient hydrated, and she clearly worked very hard for long, ten-hour days. Still, the only complaint she recorded is the occasional "do not think I learned anything new today." For Clymer, absorbing new information, becoming a new person, and finding a way to make a living trumped all the hard work.[7]

By the 1890s some American nurse leaders and their supporters began to argue for improvements in their hospital-based learning environment. Among other problems, they did not really control their schools. There was no budget for teaching, for example; usually instruction was incidental to doing the work of the hospital. In many schools admission standards were low and dictated by the number of pupils needed to meet patient care needs. Each hospital and school, unrestrained by outside interference, made up its own rules for admissions and curriculum.

But that does not mean that the nurse opinion makers and superintendents of the 1890s were calling for removing their schools from hospitals. On the contrary, they were committed to the extension of hospital school reform, to the standardization of the curriculum and management of their schools and hospitals, and perhaps most of all, to the improvement of their own authority within their institutions.

Nursing Perspectives in the Late Nineteenth Century

We can get a sense of the thinking of nursing leaders from the papers given at the 1893 Columbian Exposition or World's Fair in Chicago. The nursing sessions of the International Congress of Charities, Corrections, and Philanthropy were organized by Isabel Hampton (later Robb), of Johns Hopkins Hospital in Baltimore, and Englishwoman Ethel Bedford Fenwick. They included papers from a wide array of nurse innovators and leaders. Historians now see the 1893 meeting as something of a "coming-out party" for organized nursing in the United States. Here Isabel Hampton called for the preparation of an "intelligent saint" who will be loyal to what she is taught. Hampton argued for work as education and exalted the school's responsibility to the hospital. Lavinia L. Dock, also from Johns Hopkins, maintained that to staff the hospital with fully trained, graduate nurses would, in addition to being too costly, risk loss of control because fully trained nurses would have their own ideas about how to nurse. Dock favored a military model of hospital organization. A paper from Florence Nightingale argued that a well-organized hospital was the best basis for teaching the nurse to help the patient. She went on to warn that relying on books and lectures as a means for learning to nurse was the greatest danger of all. And she added a strong plea for creating homes for nurses led by morally strong superintendents to counter the danger of what she called "a life of freedom" for graduate nurses. All in all, the tone in 1893 was conservative and authoritarian.

The Visiting Nurse

I come back to the turn of the twentieth century later in this chapter, but now I want to turn to another nineteenth-century reform in health care, the invention of the "visiting nurse." Every town and city in the rapidly growing United States struggled with the problems posed by destitute people who became sick or disabled. Elderly people without family help also became a public responsibility. Almshouses and so-called poor farms offered meager shelter and food but little or nothing in the way of health care. Benevolent citizens organized themselves to help, sometimes in the form of women making "friendly visits" to the poor and elderly in their homes.

The problem of the poor and the public response to their plight was, of course, complicated and influenced by morally grounded beliefs about the reasons for their condition. Were they poor because they were depraved? Or were they depraved because they were poor? What was the moral responsibility of the citizen, the family, and the community for these people? In one area general agreement can be found. Unhealthy people, especially those with infectious diseases such as tuberculosis, typhoid, smallpox, dysentery, and scarlet fever, posed a danger to the larger community. So the option of doing nothing was obviated by fear of contamination.

The earliest prototype of the visiting nurse was created by the Ladies Benevolent Society of Charleston, South Carolina, in 1813, when Charleston was blockaded by the British during the War of 1812. The ladies attended to the sick in their homes, offering food and medicine and eventually nursing care. But as historian Karen Buhler-Wilkerson notes, their example would not be replicated elsewhere until after midcentury.[8]

In the 1880s affluent women began to gather together to consider the dangers posed by the sick poor and what they could do to protect their communities. The model they chose was district nursing in England. There the first effort to send nurses into the homes of the poor was instigated by William Rathbone, a Quaker philanthropist from Liverpool. In 1859, impressed by the skill of his wife's nurse, he concluded that a nurse could not only care for the sick at home but also help them learn to care for themselves. Seeking more nurses, he contacted Nightingale, who, although she was unable to help him find nurses, offered much advice and encouragement.

Rathbone founded a school to train women for the work and organized it by district, each supervised by a lady. Apparently, the district model copied Rathbone's system for dispensing relief in Liverpool.[9] Interestingly, the district model with nurse supervision by ladies was also used by Joseph Warrington to organize care for patients by his Philadelphia Nurse Society in 1839.

In 1875 Rathbone underwrote a study of district nursing, which had grown in popularity and was being replicated throughout England in the 1860s. During the fifteen years after his Liverpool experiment began, questions began to be raised about the quality and ability of the nurses in many of these replications. The study, conducted by Florence Lees, a graduate of St. Thomas', validated these concerns. Lees's recommendations included providing more education for the district nurse, recruiting higher-class women for district nursing, and supplying respectable and supportive homes for district nurses. It was this reformed pattern of district nursing that was copied by American philanthropists. Rathbone and Lees's improved model influenced the creation of visiting nurse societies in New York, Chicago, Philadelphia, Boston, Buffalo, and eventually cities all across the United States.

Nightingale's Influence

Throughout this period Nightingale was writing letters and articles about the district nursing movement. The public learned of district nursing through Nightingale's letter to *The Times*, "Untrained Nursing for the Sick Poor."[10] Nightingale believed in the importance and efficacy of nursing in the home, and she had a clear vision of what it should be. But the heavy lifting to make it happen depended on Rathbone and Lees, who built the model and implemented it. In this sense, the district nursing story helps us develop our picture of how Nightingale fits into the larger story of the invention of modern nursing.

For Americans, especially those seeking to carve out a new kind of nursing and new work for women, Nightingale's celebrity and name recognition served to brand modern nursing in a palatable way. Among the many nineteenth-century examples of this link was the "Florence Nightingale Pledge," written by a committee chaired by Lystra E. Gretter, principal of the Farrand Training School for Nurses in Detroit. Gretter's 1893 pledge was modeled after the Hippocratic Oath used by physicians and similarly intended to guarantee that the public could trust the modern trained nurse. The pledge emphasized purity, faithful professionalism, confidentiality, loyalty to the physician, and devotion to the patient. I wonder if the aging Nightingale would have approved, but of course her name no longer belonged to her. For Americans, she was a remote figure in faraway England whose image would be cast and recast in appealing ways.

So for late nineteenth- and early twentieth-century nursing leaders seeking expanded authority and power-engendering respectability, the mythical image of Nightingale as a self-sacrificing humanitarian from the upper echelons of English society was irresistible. In the same way, American physicians made a legend out of William Osler, who embodied their longing to be seen as brilliant clinical thinkers who could be trusted to put the patient's interests first.[11] Through these legends both medicine and nursing strove to create an enhanced identity and status within the culture that would support their claims as professions.

Rejecting Nightingale

At the same time, though, American nurses completely ignored or rejected Nightingale's views on two central aspects of health care and professional development. These are, of course, the acceptance of the germ theory of disease causation and the education, registration, and licensure of nurses.

Germs

It seems that Nightingale resisted the idea that disease could be random and induced by a specific contagion. Until the 1880s most Americans shared her belief in a more general atmospheric source of infection, that is, a miasma. But as Louis Pasteur and later Robert Koch began to show that certain microbes were associated with specific diseases, people started to take interest in germ theory. As historian Nancy Tomes explains in *The Gospel of Germs,* people were eager for some way to reduce their fear of infectious diseases.[12] Tuberculosis and the growing movement to fight it raised public consciousness about germs. Although germ theory offered nothing in the way of cure, it did seem to offer a route to prevention. Public health measures to clean and protect water supplies, regulate handling of milk, and other sanitary reforms found support through the growing public belief in this new way of understanding the transmission of disease.

But for Nightingale, disease emanated from dirt, disorder, and a contaminated atmosphere. To deny this, she believed, would weaken hospital reforms and undermine the need for hospitals. Her initial opposition, though, was more fundamental than that. In his essay "Florence Nightingale on Contagion: The Hospital as Moral Universe," Charles Rosenberg lays out her views, which were shared by many in the mid-nineteenth century.[13] For her, the body was seen as in a dynamic, constant interaction with the environment. Health was equated with balance within that environment, and disease was seen as a general state of imbalance. Others would begin to shift their views to assume that most diseases had a specific cause, but Nightingale was reluctant to do so. Everything she believed about nursing and hospitals or care of the sick in their homes rested on, as Rosenberg puts it, "morally resonant polarities: filth as opposed to purity, order versus disorder, health in contradistinction to disease."[14] And thus the task of the nurse must be to put the patient in the best condition for nature to cure him. If disease was caused by germs attacking in an arbitrary way, then for Nightingale, the moral basis for nursing was destroyed and sickness lost its meaning. Nightingale maintained her objections to germ theory until the late 1870s or 1880s.[15]

Meanwhile, the spread of hospitals and nursing schools in the United States accelerated, as we have seen, in the 1880s and 1890s, at the same time as germ theory was gradually accepted. Nurses in the hospital were charged with the tasks of maintaining not only order but cleanliness. Segregation of patients with infectious diseases and the nurses who cared for them grew to be common. Disinfection of operating rooms, maternity wards, and hospital equipment were seen as essential to the successful hospital. American nurses began to wear white uniforms in the late 1890s to symbolize this emphasis on safe, antiseptic caretaking. The risks they took via their exposure to patients with infectious diseases were high; they tried to protect themselves as best they could. But their understanding of the idea of contagion from germs did not, as Nightingale feared, destroy either nursing or the hospital.

Education, Registration, and Licenses

In the United States the habit of forming self-supporting, voluntary interest groups dates to the founding of the country. Nurses certainly embraced the idea of organizing, especially as their numbers grew, as they did from the 1890s forward. In 1900 there were 12,026 trained nurses listed in the census. By 1910 there were 82,327, more than six times as many.

The 1893 nursing sessions at the Chicago World's Fair helped stimulate this tendency to organize. It brought Isabel Hampton, Lavinia Dock, and Ethel Bedford Fenwick together. Fenwick, an early supporter and instigator of the British Nurses Association in 1887, encouraged Hampton, Dock, and others to move forward. They organized the American Society of Superintendents of Training Schools for Nurses that same year. During the 1890s American nurses who had trained in various hospitals began to band together in alumnae associations. Though each alumnae group reflected the ethnic and religious orientation of its hospital, they began to affiliate with local, state, and national associations of nurses. The alumnae association groups banded together in 1896 to create what became the American Nurses Association in 1911.

The agenda for all these associations was ambitious. They planned higher educational standards for incoming nursing students, proposed a preliminary course of instruction before students took care of patients, advocated a uniform curriculum, and wanted to extend the training program to three years. Beginning in about 1900, what Dock called "progressive" nurse superintendents tried to improve their schools by establishing a probationary period for every new pupil, teaching a standard curriculum with set times for each subject, hiring instructors with postgraduate education, and setting higher standards for admission. Of course, this effort was a struggle because these improvements cost money. The larger schools made faster progress, and at many meetings smaller schools were criticized for failing to adopt these twentieth-century reforms.

The crucial step would be examination and registration of nurses by the states. Each state would certify or register hospital-trained nurses the same way it licensed physicians and would make it illegal for untrained competitors to invoke the title of trained or registered nurse.

American nurse leaders viewed registration as essential to elevating the status of their profession and the prestige of women. They saw it in much the same way as they viewed the vote for women. And they went to work on the project right away. For instance, in Pennsylvania, alumnae groups banded together and organized the Pennsylvania Nurses Association in 1903. A draft bill to propose legislation was ready by 1904 and introduced to the legislature by 1905. After many efforts and compromises a registration bill was passed in 1909 and a state board to oversee professional nursing was established.

The registration movement was successful in that nurses were able to secure laws overseeing entrance into the profession in almost every state. But registration laws were often weak and almost always included a "grandfather clause" that allowed those already practicing nursing when the law was passed to continue. Three decades would pass before more stringent registration control was exerted over entry into the nursing labor force.

Nightingale apparently never made any public statements about registration, but her views on evaluating nurses were well known. She did not believe any kind of written test could verify a nurse's ability. Her vision of nursing was one of character and witnessed competence. She was adamant that nursing remain distinct from medicine. As noted above, she wrote to the 1893 gathering that relying on books and lectures to teach nurses was the greatest danger of all. Nightingale insisted that nurse training be practical and ward-based. She strongly disapproved of Rebecca Strong's much-admired preliminary training program at the Glasgow Royal Hospital, where new pupils received instruction before caring for patients. According to Anne Marie Rafferty, Nightingale worried that certification would act as an alternative to improving one-self as a woman and a nurse.[16] She believed nursing to be essentially a private act, not a field of work to be tested in the public sector.

What is so interesting about these significant differences between American nurses and Nightingale is that they were never mentioned in any of the thousands of words American nurses wrote about Nightingale. And even now her early objections to the germ theory of disease, her views on education, and her negative views on certification and licensure receive little or no attention. It seems that American nurses cheerfully ignored Nightingale when it suited them.

American Views of Nightingale

When Nightingale died in August 1910, eulogies appeared in many major American newspapers, including the *New York Times*. The *Times* account was detailed, offering a chronology of her life, including, of course, her heroic days in the Crimea. Then the account claimed that Nightingale originally wanted to be a physician and when frustrated in this goal set out to open the professions to women. Of course, in reality Nightingale did neither. The *Times* next asserted that Nightingale fought for women's suffrage, which she did not.[17] This seems to me to be another, more general example of using Florence Nightingale to exhort for popular causes, notwithstanding the facts of her life.

In 1939 Adelaide Nutting, a famous American nurse educator, was invited to speak at a gathering where a recording of Nightingale's voice was being promoted for sale. Nutting was the honorary chair of the Florence Nightingale International Foundation, founded in 1934. The Nightingale recording was part of the Edison project; it had been made in 1890 by Thomas Edison and then restored with 1930s technology.[18] Nutting used the occasion to cite Nightingale's contributions; she focused on Nightingale's faith in education as the only way to remedy the ills of humankind. She went on to credit Nightingale as the sole founder of district nursing. Then she detailed the many contributions of schools of nursing and explained the debt American society owed to the schools for the nation's advances in health. Those familiar with Nutting's writing and speeches recognize that she was putting her own words in Nightingale's mouth. In fact, as the first holder (in 1907) of a professor's chair at Columbia University in New York City, Nutting was the personification of

Nightingale's fear that nursing would be drawn into the university and lose its moral footing and special character.

So it seems that for Americans, Nightingale could be Longfellow's "Lady with a Lamp" and she could be Nutting's "brain cutting like a Damascus blade through the immaterial."[19] Most of all, she remains a malleable, mythical, historic figure. And when it suits us, we are not reluctant, notwithstanding historical fact, to use an abstract, vague, even untrue vision of Nightingale if it can help us enhance our own beliefs and protect and even enforce our own values. We think we know who she was. In all probability, however, most Americans do not. Given her impact on our world, this gives us all the more reason to reexamine this amazing woman of the nineteenth century one hundred years after her death.

MYTHOLOGIZING AND DE-MYTHOLOGIZING

LYNN MCDONALD

Historians in recent decades have delighted in "de-mythologizing" Florence Nightingale, who was a legend in her lifetime and who attracted an unholy amount of hagiographical commentary, although always with opposition and no little amount of sexism. A major source of this "de-mythologizing" is an article published in 1985 by the distinguished nursing historian Monica Baly, "The Nightingale Nurses: The Myth and the Reality." Baly in turn was influenced by F. B. Smith's vitriolic and highly inaccurate *Florence Nightingale: Reputation and Power.*[1] Numerous other academics followed in their footsteps, adding nothing from research on primary sources but rather embellishing Baly and Smith's points.[2]

The result has been the emergence of a "re-mythologized" Nightingale, now condemned for an extraordinary list of failings, from personal character (with accusations of stealing nurses' material) to incompetence and negligence (including the high death rates at the Crimean War, neglect of her own training school, and failure to guide and mentor nurses). This negative secondary literature has become for many authors a new canon, quoted as if reliable. The best biography, E. T. Cook's *The Life of Florence Nightingale,* published in 1913, is attacked as "hagiography" and therefore wrong, although it is prodigiously accurate and comprehensive in its use of original sources. Anne Summers suggests that "serious historians" should "continue to rely" on Cook but advises that they use the book "in conjunction with" F. B. Smith's![3]

Although the de-mythologizers have presented themselves as revisionist scholars whose assiduous research has come up with new findings, in fact new findings are conspicuously absent from their publications. The two most-cited hostile sources, F. B. Smith and Hugh Small, omit major salient sources, although the authors did read some primary material. Some prominent authors did no primary research at all but rely overwhelmingly on a small number of flawed sources (notably F. B. Smith). Speculation and sarcasm are liberally used. The debate, in short, has not been one of differences of interpretation among experts working on the same body of information.

This chapter gives examples of four "myths" that have emerged ostensibly in the course of de-mythologizing that then became new myths:

1. that Nightingale was responsible for the high mortality rate in the Crimean War (some authors add that the guilt led her to have a nervous breakdown);
2. that Nightingale was a lifelong opponent of germ theory;
3. that Nightingale nursing amounted to mere housekeeping; and
4. that the achievements of the Nightingale School were disappointing and exaggerated.

For each one, the claim is stated, followed by excerpts from pertinent primary sources, obtained for *The Collected Works of Florence Nightingale*, that show quite the opposite.

Myth 1: Responsibility for Crimean War Deaths

Hugh Small, in *Florence Nightingale: Avenging Angel*, makes the astonishing claim that Nightingale was personally responsible for the high death rate in the Barrack Hospital at Scutari and felt so guilty as a result that "she suffered a complete mental and physical collapse" on her return to England. Although she had been proud of her achievements on her return in 1856, he suggests, by 1857 she had discovered the "proof," the "real reason" for the loss of the army. "She suffered a complete mental and physical collapse," and her "illness," which he puts in quotation marks, began.[4]

Small's book was enthusiastically endorsed, "a must read for seekers of truth in knowledge," "an exciting revelation" of how "Nightingale discovered her culpability" in the deaths of soldiers. "She broke down from overwhelming guilt."[5] The *Sunday Times* is even more succinct in its story: "Under her nursing supervision during the Crimean war, hundreds of wounded soldiers died unnecessarily."[6]

Small's conclusions have been taken up with gusto by other authors and were featured in two BBC broadcasts: a BBC2 "documentary" in 2001, in which he took part, and a BBC1 "docudrama" in 2008, which he claims plagiarized his book. (The director of that film had only flimsy excuses for the coincidences.) The nervous breakdown of the book is renamed in the BBC film a "spiritual and emotional breakdown."

The *Sunday Times* story on the film is an unrelieved attack whereas the film shows both positives and negatives. The story asserts that Nightingale was "unwittingly responsible for 5000 unnecessary deaths." "Overcome by remorse," she took to her bed, the story goes, but her father's guidance helped her to recover, a speculation initially suggested by Small.[7] Small's "evidence" effectively amounts to surmises about missing correspondence, however, and the BBC offers none at all. Given that Nightingale's father thwarted her work for years before the Crimean War and took no interest in it afterward, the case seems unlikely.

Clive Ponting repeats with conviction many of the points made by F. B. Smith and Hugh Small in a book that puts both "myth" and "truth" in the title: *The Crimean War: The Truth behind the Myth*.[8] Yet he cites no primary sources on Nightingale. Ponting further claims that the sanitary situation of the hospital where she worked was good before she arrived (citing the biographer of Sidney Herbert, a highly interested party, and a position contrary to Herbert's own). Ponting concludes that Nightingale "achieved very little," and without taking into account any differences in the conditions of the hospitals or of their patients, he maintains that under her "the death rate at Scutari remained far higher than that of the front-line hospitals in Balaclava."[9] Ponting correctly points out that the sanitary commission that was finally sent out improved things, but he sees those improvements as "an indictment of the previous management (including that of Florence Nightingale)." This is an odd point given that the two surviving members of that commission, John Sutherland and Robert Rawlinson, became Nightingale's lifelong collaborators. They clearly did not believe that she was responsible for the appalling death rates.

Nightingale in fact was not having any sort of nervous, emotional, or spiritual breakdown post-Crimea, but was busy documenting the causes of the disaster and devising structural changes to ensure that they would never recur. With a team of public health experts, she succeeded in getting a royal commission established to do an official inquiry, for which she did much of the background work. That much at least is well recognized. That she also gave some two years of her life to researching and writing up a more substantial document is not. The request came from Lord Panmure, the war minister. It was to be a "précis," to be ready in six months. It turned out to be a nine-hundred-page analysis of what went wrong and took close to two years: *Notes on Matters Affecting the Health, Efficiency and Hospital Administration of the British Army Founded Chiefly on the Experience of the Late War* (hereafter *Matters Affecting*).[10] When the War Office made available the official correspondence throughout the war, Nightingale excerpted it for a lengthy appendix in the official report, Appendix LXXIX, consisting of 976 items in seven sections. She drew on these for her "confidential report," interspersing them with her analysis. The excerpts (in both documents) show that doctors in the field sent in reports of problems from the landing of the troops in Bulgaria, before the war started, through the move to the battlefield and the horrors of the Barrack Hospital at Scutari.

Keith Williams, remarkably for an article published in 2008 (albeit from an ongoing doctoral dissertation), believes that hostile comments have been few and recent and that the "popular image" of Nightingale remains "the angel of Scutari" and "the genius" behind "much medical reform and the development of nursing."[11] This reputation he calls the product of "myth," and he argues that "far from guiding the reform and development of military medicine," "she did more harm than good," according to "much evidence," although he includes no such evidence in support.

Williams takes Nightingale to task, as have many commentators, for her criticism of the inspector general of hospitals, Dr. John Hall, notably for her rude remarks on his being made a KCB (Knight Commander of the Bath). In private correspondence she renamed his title "Knight of the Crimean Burial-grounds." Yet Williams fails to mention the reasons Nightingale thought Hall undeserving, which are set out in detail in *Matters Affecting*.

Briefly, Lord Raglan, commander-in-chief, sent Hall out to inspect the Barrack Hospital at Scutari, and he gave it a glowing report, which he stuck to even as doctors' reports came in that said otherwise. Defects in the Barrack Hospital sewers were reported as early as 4 August 1854, before Nightingale was even appointed superintendent of nursing. Privies were "in disrepair and contaminating the atmosphere in that part of the building, endangering the health of the troops there." Pipes burst with filth, so that the ground floor was "covered with filth in consequence," while the main sewer was obstructed. Nothing was done to repair the structural defects, and in London Dr. Andrew Smith, director general of the Army Medical Department, left the matter for five months before he inquired.

Hall's report of 20 October 1854 to Smith expressed "much satisfaction in being able to inform him that the whole hospital establishment here (at Scutari) has now been put on a very creditable footing, and that the sick and wounded are all doing as well as could possibly be expected." "All our difficulties" had been "in great measure surmounted," he reported. Lord Raglan was also taken in by the "flourishing account" Hall sent.[12] The Duke of Newcastle, the senior war minister, evidently was not promptly apprised of the negative reports. Later, when the "misery existing in the hospitals" was under investigation, he explained that problems that were identified had been denied by the Army Medical Department (in London).[13]

Williams attributes a "particular animus" against Smith on Nightingale's part, on account of his "lowly background"—his father was a shepherd.[14] Moreover, she had a general "class-based hostility to military doctors," many of whom came from humble Scots and Irish origins. Yet as *Matters Affecting* abundantly shows, she defended them and blamed the senior administrators—John Hall in the East and Andrew Smith in London—for failure to take action on the doctors' reports. Williams, reasonably enough, calls for more research in primary sources, but he seems to be unaware of the wholehearted support Nightingale gave to the ordinary military doctors, who conscientiously sent in reports to their superiors on the lack of supplies and medicine and miserable conditions endured by the soldiers during the Crimean War.

The ventilation of the Barrack Hospital was another serious defect in Nightingale's lengthy report. The "hospital," of course, had never been built as one, but rather was a barrack. A central courtyard kept the bad air in (no cross-ventilation was possible). Space per patient was one-quarter of the normal, even for a military hospital. As Nightingale stated in *Matters Affecting*:

> The buildings were spacious and magnificent in external appearance, far
> more so indeed than any military buildings in Great Britain, and several

of them were, apparently, better suited for hospitals than any military hospitals at home. This merely external appearance was, however, fatally deceptive. Underneath these great structures were sewers of the worse possible construction, loaded with filth, mere cesspools, in fact, through which the wind blew sewer air up the pipes of numerous open privies into the corridors and wards where the sick were lying.

The wards had no means of ventilation, the walls required constant lime-washing, and the number of sick crowded into the hospitals during the winter of 1854–55 was disproportionately large, especially when the bad sanitary state of the buildings is taken into consideration. The population of the hospitals was increased not only without any sanitary precautions having been taken, but while the sanitary conditions were becoming daily worse, for the sewers were getting more and more dangerous and the walls more and more saturated with organic matter.[15]

The disaster at Scutari made Nightingale skeptical about the desirability of large hospitals ever after. The Barrack Hospital housed 2,500 patients, far more than even the largest London hospitals (St. Bartholomew's had 650 at the time, St. Thomas' only 200). Nightingale wrote, "Our general hospitals have been so deplorably mismanaged in all our wars that the question has been raised as to whether it would not be better to do without them altogether. The experience of Scutari proves that general hospitals may become pest houses from neglect, or may be made as healthy as any other buildings."[16] She would pursue this idea in *Notes on Hospitals* after the war.

In contrast with the Barrack Hospital at Scutari, the Castle Hospital at Balaclava was small, located on a height, with sea breezes blowing in. The General Hospital at Balaclava was also small and had some of its sick and wounded spread out in well-ventilated huts. Other sick and wounded were placed in tents, again in small numbers. The hospitals, in short, were not at all comparable. De-mythologizers, however, have blithely taken the different results by hospital without any recognition of the sharply different conditions.

Nightingale was utterly consistent in her assessment of blame for the Crimean War debacle. In 1856, only just back home from the war, she told Sir John McNeill "that the men in authority over us" were "perfectly aware of the truth of the manslaughter committed in 1854, and of the falsehood as well as incompetency of those principally concerned in it."[17]

The next year, to family friend Christian von Bunsen, she described her work toward reform of the army as "hopeless":

> Everyone is well aware that, if war were to break out tomorrow, we should have the whole scene of '54 over again.
>
> Those who helped to lose that magnificent army are now careless, at their ease, indifferent or triumphant. Those who helped to save it are cast aside, rejected and despised.... England is a country which learns by experiments and not by experience, and she has learnt nothing by her colossal calamity. What that calamity was I believe one must have been in the Crimea to know. The newspapers were *temperate*.[18]

Writing later to a nurse in Australia about the bad conditions at the Sydney Hospital, she said that the Scutari hospitals, when she first arrived, were "slaughterhouses."[19]

Numerous further examples could be cited. Small's conclusion of self-blame is pure speculation, augmented by copious references to destroyed letters and "repression," neither of which can be refuted, for either Nightingale was not conscious of her feelings or she was and destroyed the evidence. His elaborate surmise has been enthusiastically repeated by reviewers of his book and other authors, and then taken up, without attribution, by the BBC. None of those who use his argument have taken the trouble to consult the relevant primary sources, and of course what was written in the missing letters remains unknown.

Myth 2: Lifelong Opposition to Germ Theory

Incorrect statements about Nightingale's views on germ theory are both numerous and extreme. Says a reviewer of F. B. Smith's *Florence Nightingale: Reputation and Power*: "She was most consistent where she was most wrong, as in her hostility to germ theory and her attachment to 'miasma.'" This reviewer even convicts her of causing serious harm: "No one did more to keep cholera alive and well than Nightingale."[20]

That historians of all ilks have been just as far off base can be seen in a few examples. A nursing historian states: "Contagion was the basis of what later became germ theory—a theory which Florence Nightingale, and many other social reformers, found unpalatable because it conflicted with their social agenda. Nightingale had still not accepted germ theory at the time of her death in 1910 despite its widespread acceptance."[21] According to Robert Dingwall, Anne Marie Rafferty, and Charles Webster, Nightingale "clung ferociously to miasmatic theory...long past its discrediting in the medical world."[22] Another view has Nightingale as a "dogmatic miasmatist" who remained "unsympathetic" to germ theory, even to "the end of her life."[23] In the introduction to his edition of *Notes on Hospitals,* Charles Rosenberg faults Nightingale for "her certainty" and "strident and uncompromising" views on germ theory. Her "explicit rejection" of the theory took her gradually "further apart from the consensus of medical opinion during the last third of the nineteenth century."[24] In another publication he describes Nightingale as "unwilling to accept the specificity of disease and the possible existence of specific causative agents."[25]

When Nightingale began her work in the 1850s, germ theory was no more than academic speculation. Louis Pasteur made his important breakthroughs in the 1860s, but these were on vineyard and silkworm diseases. English surgeon Joseph Lister then began to speculate that there might be parallels between Pasteur's germs and the causes of infection in surgical wounds. (Might one note a coincidence? Lister's father was a wine merchant.) In 1867 Lister, who had still not seen a germ, hypothesized that it was not the oxygen or other gaseous constituents in the air that caused putrefaction in wounds and high death rates from major surgery. Rather, "minute organisms suspended" in the air were responsible. He could identify no specific germ and hence called them "septic" or "atmospheric" germs and "floating particles." Carbolic acid was the remedy, the most powerful antiseptic then available.[26]

Germ theory made much headway after Lister. German bacteriologist Robert Koch identified anthrax in 1877 and went on to write his famous paper, "The Etiology of Traumatic Infectious Diseases," in 1879. This work is often taken to be the definitive demonstration of germ theory.

The fundamental difference between the old miasma, or environmental, theory and germ theory is that the latter specified a single disease cause, a specific bacillus, whereas miasma theory allowed multiple diseases to arise from the same miasm. With the benefit of hindsight we would explain the fact of multiple diseases arising from the same foul water as due to the existence of a multiple (different) bacilli in it. The same feces-contaminated water might cause cholera, dysentery, and diarrhea. Swamps infested with mosquitoes could produce both malaria and yellow fever.

Nightingale may never have looked into a microscope, but her colleague Dr. Sutherland did, and he brought her the crucial information about germ theory in 1884. He had been impressed with Koch's "discovery" of the cholera bacillus in a cholera epidemic in Calcutta. (The bacillus had been seen before but not persuasively shown to be the causal agent of cholera.)

Even after coming around to germ theory, however, Nightingale continued to stress practice over theory, "cleanliness first." For her time, this was sound advice, for the acceptance of germ theory brought with it no advances in treatment. Nightingale's methods were excellent at prevention, even before she corrected her theory. Baly explains how well her ideas suited: "The new sanitary ward of her dream fitted well with the germ theory when it was validated. It was easier to practise asepsis in a clean, airy, tiled ward than in the old style ward with closed windows, wooden floors and porous walls."[27]

Although the de-mythologizers would have Nightingale to be antiscientific, even impeding progress in practice, there is plenty of evidence to the contrary. By 1864 she was convinced of the value of examining water sources by microscope for problems, although without yet conceiving that the harmful substances were living germs. A report that she and John Sutherland drafted specifies how water should be allowed to settle "in a scrupulously clean glass vessel for six or eight hours, and the sediment carefully collected and examined under the microscope." For small quantities of sediment, they specified the use of a "clean conical glass vessel," the water to be "allowed to stand for three or four hours. The sediment should then be submitted to the microscope."[28] This was in fact how Koch discovered the cholera bacillus some decades later and how Nightingale herself would be convinced of the existence of microscopic disease germs.

Nightingale's insistence on preventive measures, far from impeding progress, meshed with the best practice. Indeed, the Nightingale School began teaching a rudimentary form of germ theory as early as 1873. Medical instructor John Croft's (printed) lectures to the probationers include the chapter "Disinfectants and Antiseptics," which describes the available antiseptics and their preferred uses. It ends with the admonition that antiseptics were not substitutes for ventilation, fresh air, and cleanliness, Nightingale's point precisely.[29]

Nightingale's advice on practice evolved. Simple cleanliness was the focus in her 1860 *Notes on Nursing* (pre–germ theory), but by the time she worked on the nursing article for Richard Quain's *Dictionary of*

Medicine (written in 1878, published in 1883), she had detailed advice to give, with precise quantities of the various antiseptics and disinfectants required (on which more below).

By 1891 Nightingale was so convinced of the usefulness of germ theory that she advocated its demonstration in village lectures in India. The nasty germs would be shown by slides, "a magic lantern show." She suggested to the public health organization in Pune: "Probably the village school rooms might be utilized for the lectures, which might be made attractive by object lessons, with the magic lantern showing the noxious living organisms in foul air and water."[30]

That the great Russian microbiologist Waldemar Mordecai Haffkine sought an introduction to Nightingale when he was in London in 1895 entirely fits. Sir Henry Acland was the intermediary, but there is no evidence that any such meeting took place. Acland's pitch to Nightingale was Haffkine's work on cholera in India.[31] Haffkine won the Nobel Prize in Medicine in 1908 for his work on plague and cholera.

Myth 3: Nightingale Nursing Merely "Applied Housekeeping"

F. B. Smith is firm that Nightingale's nursing amounted to mere "common sense care," that "she added nothing to the details of technical proficiency required in a nurse's daily tasks." According to Smith, "the practice of nursing was never among Miss Nightingale's prime concerns," which were "patronage and surveillance of nurses' lives." She failed to guide their professional work.[32] The final damning sentence in his chapter on nursing is, "Miss Nightingale served the cause of nursing less than it served her."[33] A reviewer of the book embellishes these points, claiming that Nightingale "lacked any originality of thought," while her "nursing never became more than a form of applied housekeeping," a view she supposedly "retained all her life."[34]

It is quite correct that the first probationers at the Nightingale School were kept to a limited number of tasks and greatly exploited by the hospital. Nightingale frequently protested their use for "drudgery" and never satisfactorily stopped it. Nurses in the first years were not allowed to take a patient's temperature, the prerogative of medical students and surgeons' assistants. It should be remembered that some doctors at the time were opposed to nurse training at all, and many were uncertain as to how much the nurses could do, given their poor education. There was no minimal educational requirement for entry, and few candidates would have applied if there had been. Remedial reading had to be provided for a long time. But Nightingale believed in starting small and not waiting for better conditions. Nevertheless, even the minimal list of duties of 1860 goes far beyond mere "housekeeping" or "common sense care."

The skills required of nurses quickly increased. The following expectations were set out in the rules for probationers when the school opened in 1860:

> You are expected to become skillful in the dressing of blisters, burns, sores, wounds and in applying fomentations, poultices and minor dressings; in the application of leeches, externally and internally; in the administration of enemas for men and women; in the management of trusses and appliances in uterine complaints; in the best method of friction to the body and extremities; in the management of helpless patients, i.e., moving, changing, personal cleanliness of, feeding, keeping warm (or cool), preventing and dressing bedsores, managing position of; in bandaging, making bandages and rollers, lining of splints, etc. . . . to attend at operations; to cook . . . ; to understand ventilation . . . by night as well as by day; you are to be careful that great cleanliness is observed in all the utensils . . . to make strict observation of the sick in the following particulars: the state of secretions, expectoration, pulse, skin, appetite, intelligence, as delirium or stupor, breathing, sleep, state of wounds, eruptions, formation of matter, effect of diet or of stimulant and of medicines; and to learn the management of convalescents.[35]

Further skills were required two decades later, as described in Nightingale's article "Nursing the Sick" in Quain's *Dictionary of Medicine*. "The physician also requires the nurse to be able to 'take' and to record the temperature," sometimes every quarter of an hour in critical cases. The taking and testing of urine was added. There is a note that observation had to be still more accurate for child patients, "who cannot tell what is the matter with them." Nurses must be able to "understand the management of sick children and children's wards, which need a yet more exquisite cleanliness. And children show a much more rapid change of symptoms for life or for death generally than adults. Children are the best air test, the best test of sanitary conditions."[36]

Moreover, nurses had to be able to pass the catheter, at least for women. "The district nurse is often now required to pass the speculum for women, also the catheter for men, because there is no one else to do it."[37] There was more detail on fomentations, poultices, and minor dressings, wet and dry or greasy; and the nurse had to be able to syringe wounds and the vagina. To the requirements for bed-making specifics were added different types of cases: fever, accidents, ovariotomy, and various kinds of operations; and the ability to undress, handle, and put to bed accident cases.[38]

Instead of merely attending at operations, the nurse had "to prepare patients for and manage them after operations and anesthetics—and all this with the least call upon their small strength." In case of hemorrhage, the nurse had to be able to apply "compression by hand or finger, by extemporary tourniquet and plugging." There was more detail about bandaging and the making of bandages.[39]

Although nurses at first did not give injections, now "the nurse should be able to give subcutaneous injections, to use the galvanic battery . . . to give inhalations and use the spray disperser; to apply cold, with the use of siphons and with ice, and antiseptic treatment." Every surgeon and physician had his own "antiseptic solutions," his own "disinfectants," and every year brought fresh ones. "And what is ordered must of course be used by the nurse."[40]

The Quain's article gives detailed instructions about the use of disinfectants; carbolic is mentioned eighteen times, with strengths of solution ranging from 1 in 20 to 1 in 100. Where disinfection would not suffice, burning was required:

> Steeping in boiling water with an antiseptic solution (carbolic acid 1 in 100) is the only safe method of disinfection. All washing of dirty linen and bandages should be done outside of the sick room and, if possible, of the house. In a hospital the laundry should be in a separate building.
>
> *Bandages* with pus on them are always to be burnt at once—to be carried straight to the ward fire, or to a furnace. The best economy is to burn them, but one must make up the fire so that the burning shall not smell. Bandages used for fractures, etc., are the only bandages that may be washed. Soak these with chlorinated soda, a diluted pint, then boil them all night with soft soap, soda and chlorinated soda—a quart bottle for the two. The bandages are then to be rinsed in a tub. The boiler must, of course, only be emptied in a closet sink.[41]

Applied housekeeping indeed!

In the 1894 edition of Quain's *Dictionary* Nightingale added a point about the need to keep improving practice: "Nursing is, above all, a progressive calling. Year by year nurses have to learn new and improved methods, as medicine and surgery and hygiene improve. Year by year nurses are called upon to do more and better than they have done."[42]

In 1896 Nightingale learned about aseptic methods from a Finnish nurse, Ellen Ekblom, and had the material printed for circulation in the school. She began to ask questions about operating theater procedures. Notes from an interview with E. L. Froude, then the operating theater sister, record: "Boiling all dressings, all bandages, aseptic in wards, handing instruments, cyanide gauze, sponges of cellulosic thrown away.... Scrubbing hands well with green soft soap and particularly one's nails; then if... any little roughness, take off with perchloride and rinse in sterilized water. We use no other in the theatre. The surgeons do the same. They like to take the instruments from perfectly clean hands."[43] Another note explains that all the pictures in the surgical wards were taken down after spring cleaning, in order to be aseptic.[44]

Also in 1896 Nightingale met with St. Thomas'–trained Helen Shuter, after her election as matron of the City of Dublin Hospital. The notes record Shuter's discontent with operating theater practices there. Apart from noting that cocaine was the only anesthetic used, Shuter called the theater "most *objectionable*." It had "none of the other theatres' improvements, wooden floor, dirty couch, nothing of the aseptic about it—no cleanliness, next door to the Out-Patients Department."[45]

Nor should Nightingale's general holistic approach to health care be mistaken for mere housekeeping. Nightingale carefully separated the role of the doctor, who was scientifically trained when women were not, from that of the nurse. But the distinctive role played by the nurse in healing was a noble one. After all, medicine does not cure, Nightingale held; healing is done by God or nature. As she described the process in the Quain's article, and repeated in 1892 for an entry on hospitals in *Chambers's Encyclopaedia*, "Nursing is putting us in the best possible conditions for nature to restore or to preserve health—to prevent or to cure disease or injury. The physician or surgeon prescribes these conditions—the nurse carries them out."[46] The doctor had to determine the medicines, diet, regime, and so on to be followed. But the nurse was responsible for their administration and for feedback to the doctor on progress, and of course the nurse was with the patient far more.

Evolving practice can also be seen in Nightingale's work on midwifery nursing. She had had to give up the midwifery nurse training at King's College Hospital as a result of an unacceptably high rate of puerperal fever. For decades thereafter she sought a way to restart this training, in a safer, that is, nonhospital, setting. Workhouse infirmaries had lower rates of death, even though the women delivering, the destitute, were less healthy. The rates were lower still for women giving birth at home. Puerperal fever is one of the rare diseases with higher rates among the more privileged, presumably the result of greater medical intervention—more doctors and medical students conducting examinations and inadvertently communicating the bacillus that causes it. The bacillus was not discovered until 1902.

Nightingale's *Introductory Notes on Lying-in Institutions* argued for strict separation between birthing mothers and sick patients: "The evidence further shows that, in any new plan, infirmary wards must be kept quite detached from lying-in wards. They should be in another part of the ground and should be provided with their own furniture, bedding, utensils, stores, kitchen and attendants. The same arrangement, at least in principle, should be carried out at all existing lying-in establishments, and every case of disease should at once be removed from the lying-in wards to the infirmary and be separately attended there."[47]

Nightingale continued to make the same case for the rest of her working life. Puerperal death rates began to decline as hospitals instituted stricter sanitary precautions, but dropped to very low proportions only with the development of antibiotics in the mid-twentieth century. Practice had to be guided by informal experience.

Although Nightingale never reestablished a midwifery nurse training program, she continued to track the issue. As district nursing spread, she gave advice on how to prevent nurses from spreading puerperal fever (or other diseases) to birthing mothers. A letter in 1892 to an advocate of the "health-at-home" mission gave this advice on "monthly" nursing, or the care of the new mother and infant at home for the first month after delivery:

The *monthly* nursing of the *poor* at their own homes is one of the gravest subjects we have. Midwives do not practise it. Doctors cannot of course. Lying-in hospitals do not teach it. The uncleanliness of the bedding—a featherbed or flock bed which may not have been picked to pieces or cleaned for years and years, which may have had several lyings-in on it—is most serious for both mother and infant, is it not?

Then the personal cleanliness of the mother after lying-in, which she can't attend to herself, and which no one but a competent district nurse can attend to (as ignorance is now). Then there is nothing about cleanliness of the *bottle* for hand fed infants in that nice little leaflet.[48]

Similarly, she advised that the matron on inspection should "go to the lying-in wards first thing in the morning before going to the general wards, and in the evening before going to the general wards."[49]

Myth 4: Poor Achievements of Nightingale School

In "The Nightingale Nurses: The Myth and the Reality," Baly concludes: "If we examine what the Nightingale School achieved in its early years, it is in fact very little." She cites Henry Bonham Carter, secretary of the Nightingale Fund Council, as saying that there had been only two good superintendents in the first ten years.[50] But that is an understatement, for the simple reason that only two had shown their great ability in that short time. If one takes the same ten-year cohort but counts the women's full working lives, the accomplishments are impressive. In addition to Agnes Jones at the Liverpool Workhouse Infirmary and Elizabeth Torrance at the Highgate Workhouse Infirmary (the two matrons presumably considered successes), there are A. L. Pringle, at the Edinburgh Royal Infirmary and later St. Thomas' (but who was still a sister at St. Thomas' when Bonham Carter made this remark); Florence Lees, the great reformer of district nursing (who did not settle down to serious work until 1875); Jessie Lennox, of the Children's Hospital at Belfast (then just a nurse at Netley); and Rebecca Strong, matron at the Dundee Royal Infirmary and the Glasgow Royal Infirmary (again still gaining experience and not yet a matron). Lucy Osburn, matron at Sydney, presumably had not been deemed worthy enough for mention in 1870. Her early mistakes were only too much still in mind, but Osburn established professional nursing in Sydney and sent out matrons over much of Australia (see chapter 3).

The numbers produced by the Nightingale School were not large, and the dropouts, whether voluntary or not, were significant, as shown in table 5.1, constructed from the probationers' registers.[51] Critics tend to make much of these low numbers, but their significance is not obvious since the critics give no comparable data from other training schools.

Table 5.1. Nightingale School Nurses, 1860–99, Destination
after Enrollment

Destination	Tally
Appointment	Total appointed: 936
St. Thomas'	492
Other hospitals	241
Workhouse infirmaries	85
District	79
International	39
Dropped out	Total dropped out: 566
Dismissed	227
Resigned	326
Died	7
No information	6
Total students	1,502

Nor are there comparable data for the production of matrons, the main way the Nightingale School made its influence. The leaders of the school—the matron, S. E. Wardroper; the secretary of the Nightingale Fund, Henry Bonham Carter; and Nightingale herself—soon realized that it could not make its impact by sheer numbers of (ordinary) nurses produced. In 1865 a policy of training "special" or "lady" probationers was adopted, and the numbers of this category gradually increased. They paid a fee, were given additional instruction, and were exempted from some of the menial tasks. Beginning in 1868, fees were waived for persons who lacked means but were otherwise qualified.[52] By 1883, 19 specials were admitted, compared with 35 ordinary probationers; in 1890, 21 specials and 29 ordinary.

There is no lack of information on the appointment of Nightingale School former probationers as matrons, not only in Britain but in Europe, the United States, Australia, and around the world. It is hard to imagine that any other school, even the much larger London Hospital, produced more matrons and deployed them to greater effect. The list in table 5.2 shows, for the years 1860–99, the hospitals that had Nightingale School–trained matrons. The data come from the probationers' registers, augmented by death notices, obituaries, memoirs, other published sources, and correspondence obtained for *The Collected Works of Florence Nightingale*. Indication of a hospital signifies only that a matron was appointed, not how long she remained nor to what good effect, if any. The list is not an indication of the influence of Nightingale herself, for she would

Table 5.2. Hospitals with Nightingale School–Trained Matrons, 1860–99

Location	Hospitals
London	St. Thomas'; St. Mary's, Paddington; St. Bartholomew's; Westminster; Middlesex; Guy's; Charing Cross; King's College; University College; St. George's; Soho Sq. Hosp. for Women; New Hosp. for Women; Royal Hosp. for Incurables, Putney; Royal London Ophthalmic; Hosp. for Consumption, Brompton; Royal Victoria Hosp. for Children, Chelsea; Children's Hosp., Shadwell; Children's Hosp., Gt. Ormond St.; London Homeopathic; Royal Ear Hosp., Soho; Lewisham Inf.; Haverstock Hill Inf.; Shoreham Inf.; Convalescent Home for Sick Children, St. Pancras; Fulham Inf.; Homerton Fever Hosp.; Waterloo Rd. Hosp.; Harrow Rd. Hosp. for Women and Children; Isleworth Inf.
Southern England	Radcliffe Inf., Oxford; Addenbrooke's Hosp., Cambridge; Chichester Hosp.; Royal Inf.; Salisbury Inf.; Norfolk and Norwich Hosp.; Folkestone Hosp.; Sussex County Hosp.; Bristol: Royal Inf., Women's Hosp.; Royal Seabathing Hosp., Margate; Devon and Exeter Hosp.; Ipswich Hosp.; Croydon General; Smallpox Hosp., Croydon; Southend-on-Sea Sanitorium; Northampton Inf.; Brighton and Sussex Inf., Brighton and Sussex Throat and Ear; Portsmouth Hosp.; Kent and Canterbury Hosp.; East Sussex Hosp., Hastings; Babies Castle, Kent; Royal Berkshire Hosp., Reading; Royal Hampshire County Hosp.; County Hosp., Gloucester; Royal Inf., Cheltenham General; Darenth Asylum; Horton Inf.; Banbury Inf.; Halifax Inf.; Mildenhall Hosp., Suffolk; Bedfordshire Hosp.; Isolation Hosp., Wimbledon; Lowestaft Hosp.; Shrewsbury Sanitorium; Bath Eye Inf.; Taunton Somerset Hosp.; Ashton-under-Lyme Inf.; Chartham Sanatorium; Monkwearmouth Dispensary, Tetbury; Buchanan Hosp., St. Leonards; Richmond Royal Hosp.
Midlands and North	Liverpool: Royal (Southern) Inf.; Northern; Hosp. for Infectious Diseases; Mill Rd. Inf.; City Hosp., North Liverpool; Women's Hosp., Shaw St.; Children's Hosp., Myrtle St.; Manchester: Royal Inf., Ophthalmic Hosp., Heaton Mersey, Monsall Fever Hosp.; Lying-in Hosp.; Lincoln Hosp.; Royal Cumberland Inf., Carlisle; Royal Eye Hosp.; Birmingham: General Hosp., Queen's Hosp., Maternity Hosp.; Newcastle-upon-Tyne: General Hosp. and Children's Hosp.; Royal Orthopedic Hosp.; Stafford Inf.; Children's Inf., Kirkdale; Leeds: Hosp. for Women and Children, Infectious Hosp., City Hosp.; Sheffield; Pendlebury Children's Hosp.; Stoke-on-Trent Inf.; Coventry and Warwickshire Hosp.; Worcester Hosp.; Royal Northern Hosp.; Bradford Eye and Ear Hosp.; Warrington Isolation Hosp.; Blackburn Inf.; Wolverhampton Inf.; Bradford Inf.; Kidderminster Inf., Albert Inf., Cheshire; Chester General Inf.; York County Hosp.; Derby Royal Inf.; Women's Hosp., Nottingham; Salford Dispensary, Banbury; Bromsgrove and Redditch Isolation; St. Monica's Children's Hosp., Kilburn
Wales	Aberystwith Inf.; Cardiff Inf.; Swansea Inf.; Carnarvon Anglesea Inf.

(Continued)

Table 5.2. Hospitals with Nightingale School–Trained Matrons, 1860–99 (Continued)

Location	Hospitals
Scotland	Edinburgh: Royal Inf., Hosp. for Sick Children and Convalescent Home; Glasgow: Royal Inf., Western Inf.; Aberdeen: Royal Inf. and City Hosp.; Dundee Royal Inf.; Leith Hosp.; St. Andrews Hosp., Fife; Inverness Inf.; Gartlock Lunatic Asylum
Ireland	Dublin: Rotunda Hosp.; Fever Hosp.; City of Dublin Hosp.; Dr. Steevens Hosp.; Sir Patrick Duns Hosp.; Royal Hosp. for Incurables; Belfast: Children's Hosp., Lying-in Hosp., and Nightingale Nursing Home; Thompson Memorial Home, Lisburn
Military hospitals	Royal Victoria Hosp., Netley; Naval Hosp., Haslar; Royal Victoria Hosp., Bournemouth; Herbert Hosp., Woolwich; Military Fever Wards, Royal Military Inf., Dublin; Female Garrison Hosp., Portsmouth; Portsmouth Lock Hosp.; Military Isolation Hosp., Aldershot; Hosp. for Paralyzed Soldiers, Nottingham; King Edward 7th Sanitorium, Midhurst; First Eastern General Hosp.; Queen Alexandra Imperial Military Nursing Service
Workhouse infirmaries	London: Highgate; St. Marylebone, Paddington; Hampstead; Whitechapel; Holborn; Southern England: Bolton Inf.; Midlands and North: Liverpool; Birmingham; Warrington
District Nursing	Metropolitan and National District Nursing Assoc., Bloomsbury Sq. (headquarters); South London District, Battersea; Chelsea; Southwark, Newington, and Walworth District; Edgeware Rd.; East London Nursing Society; Liverpool; and numerous districts
Europe	
Sweden	Sabbatsbergs Hosp. and Sophiahemmet Nursing School, Stockholm; Uppsala University Hosp.
Germany	City Hosp., Berlin; Darmstadt Hosp. and Training School
France	Ruffi Hosp., Nimes
Finland	Helsinki: Kuopio University and Surgical Hosp.
North and South America	
United States	Boston: Massachusetts General Hosp., Waltham Training School, City Hosp., and New England Hosp. for Women and Children; Hosp. for Women and Children, Roxbury, Mass; Taunton Hosp. for the Insane, Mass.; Philadelphia: Blockley Hosp. and University of Pennsylvania; University of Maryland Hosp. and Training School, Baltimore; Salt Lake City Hosp.
Canada	Montreal General Hosp.
South America	English Hosp., Buenos Aires; English Hosp., Rio de Janeiro
West Indies	Cottage Hosp., St. Lucia; Government Hosp., St. Vincent
Australia and New Zealand	
Australia	Sydney Inf.; Alfred Hosp., Melbourne; Brisbane Inf.; Newport, Adelaide, and Perth Colonial Hosp.; Gladesville Hosp. for Insane
New Zealand	Masterton Hosp.

(Continued)

Table 5.2. Hospitals with Nightingale School–Trained Matrons, 1860–99 (Continued)

Location	Hospitals
Other	
India	Calcutta: Eden Hosp., General Hosp.; HH Nizam's Hosp., Hyderabad
Ceylon [Sri Lanka]	General Hosp., Colombo
Africa	Albany General Hosp., Grahamstown; Transvaal and Grey Hosp.; Kimberley Hosp.; King Williamstown; Government Hosp., Mafeking, Basutoland; Government Hosp., Suez; Vincent Hosp., Nigeria
Japan	Yokohama General Hosp.; Mission Hosp., Kyoto
Fiji	Suva Hosp.

have been involved in only a small portion of the appointments and she mentored only a small number of the matrons. On the other hand, the list excludes matrons who were not former pupils but for whom Nightingale acted as mentor. (Notable examples are Eva Lückes at the London Hospital, Isabel Hampton Robb and Elisabeth Robinson Scovil in the United States, and Charlotte Macleod in both the United States and Canada.) The list would be much longer still if appointments of matrons at small convalescent homes and cottage hospitals were included.

How could so many authors get it so wrong? The best source on the training and appointment of matrons is still Lucy R. Seymer's *Florence Nightingale's Nurses: The Nightingale Training School, 1860–1960,* published on the one hundredth anniversary of the founding of the school.[53] Seymer was able to take advantage of the major deposit of Nightingale papers on nursing at the British Library in 1954, which includes a massive amount of correspondence *from* matrons *to* Nightingale. She seems to have been the first nursing historian to have done so, at least thoroughly. Baly did some reading of those sources, but not as much. Moreover, Baly castigates Seymer for failing to discuss the insobriety of the medical instructor at St. Thomas'.[54] Regrettably, it seems that later nursing historians, who did not do primary research themselves, have ignored Seymer's excellent research, succinctly reported in a 169-page book. Neither F. B. Smith nor Dingwall, Rafferty, and Webster even cite this major source.

Baly's second, abbreviated, article on the "myth" theme appears on the surface to be more negative: "Shattering the Nightingale Myth."[55] But both articles give a great deal of positive information, with Baly's acerbic wit. If a myth was shattered, it would be that founding the nursing profession was unproblematic, without serious reversals and enormous trouble. But who ever said that?

Despite the negative opinions Baly has on Nightingale's nursing in general, she finds much to praise in her workhouse infirmary reforms, "first in Highgate, then at St. Marylebone, from whence the ripples spread across the pond of Poor Law nursing in general." She also flags the importance of Nightingale's work on district nursing.[56]

But F. B. Smith finds fault even with the workhouse reforms. He scorns all the hard work at Liverpool and mocks Nightingale's efforts at reform in London. She was "relegated to impotent officiousness on the workhouse question," he declares, when she did not see the legislation she sought enacted. Then the death of Agnes Jones, the pioneer of workhouse infirmary nursing in Liverpool, "rescued her."[57] Nightingale in fact was put to an enormous amount of largely futile work to replace Jones (it took years to find an adequate person). Nightingale's article "Una and the Lions" was both a tribute to Jones and a recruiting call to the intrepid to take on such tough work. Smith instead describes this as "a remarkable piece of autobiographical wish fulfillment, half-conscious projection of herself, outright mendacity and a calculated pleading."[58] But the article in fact brought in recruits, most notably F. E. Spencer, later matron of the Edinburgh Royal Infirmary.[59]

Baly's stance on Nightingale is inconsistent, to say the least. Her first publications, before she read F. B. Smith, although based only on published sources, are highly complimentary. In the first edition of *Nursing and Social Change* (1973), the chapter "The Influence of Miss Nightingale" recognizes the "legend" status of Nightingale and the "subsequent reaction of antimyth." But Baly affirms that neither could "destroy the solid fact of her achievements. They were Herculean." She credits Nightingale with having "laboured unremittingly" for fifty years, with "a first-class intellect, a passion for statistics, influence in high places…and above all the imagination to see what needed to be done." Moreover, her efforts applied not only to the "reform of nursing and hospitals, but to all aspects of the prevention of ill health in the community."[60]

Baly's doctoral research is a fine piece of work, based on a thorough investigation with significant use of primary sources.[61] But she never added to that primary research base, so that her later books, if they cite primary sources at all, give precisely the same list.

After the publication of Smith's attack on Nightingale, Baly's high praise for Nightingale's achievements is replaced by more qualified comments and later outright denigration. Compare the ringing, pre–Smith book endorsement above with the second edition of her *Florence Nightingale and the Nursing Legacy* (1985). There Baly prosaically argues that the Nightingale Fund succeeded in establishing secular nursing earlier than would otherwise have occurred. "For fifty years, with a very limited income, it managed to achieve a great deal in different spheres and because of its prestige and publicity its influence on nursing was probably out of proportion to the actual achievement in terms of nurses trained."[62]

By the third edition of *Nursing and Social Change* (1995), a new section announces: "The first ten years of the school were disastrous. Mrs. Wardroper selected working class girls who came and went with amazing rapidity."[63] Since neither the probationer's nor her father's occupation is stated, it is not evident how Baly could have drawn any inference as to social class origins. She is highly critical about the dropouts from the school, although the proportion remained about the same throughout the first fifty years, and comparable data from other schools are not available to give context. That "so many were dismissed for glaring defects like drug addiction, phthisis, syphilis and insobriety suggest that either Mrs. Wardroper's judgment was at fault or that there was no choice."[64] Again, Baly fails to show that other training schools did any better. She is sarcastic about the advertisements the Nightingale Fund Council put out. "For all its vaunted publicity the Nightingale system was not a break with the past." She refers back to the myth "that nursing suddenly became homogeneous and educated," without citing any source—whoever said that? "Under the Nightingale system undoubtedly nursing and hygiene improved. There developed a career structure for nurses," Baly allows.[65] But then she faults later nursing leaders for not having Nightingale's willingness to experiment and for retaining old requirements that were no longer needed.

Baly's last publication on Nightingale is the (posthumous) entry on her in the *Oxford Dictionary of National Biography,* an overwhelmingly negative account of Nightingale's work and person. There is no nuance left, and F. B. Smith is cited lavishly. His "striking study (1982) stripped away the iconic aspects of the Nightingale legend to examine the remarkable network of manipulation (mostly by letter) by which she sought to impose her will and achieve her objectives."[66]

Where Baly had up until then seen Nightingale's workhouse reforms as significant, here she accepts Smith's scathing account, passing off the work with a brief and grossly misleading paragraph. She acknowledges that Agnes Jones and the eight nurses sent by the Nightingale Fund to the Liverpool Workhouse Infirmary "battled against appalling conditions and prejudice." But then, following Smith, she asserts that the whole "scheme came to an end" in 1868 on Jones's death. Then, according to Baly, Nightingale "threw her influence behind the Association for Improving Workhouse Infirmaries," whose leaders Baly names as John Stuart Mill, Charles Dickens, and Louisa Twining. Nightingale in fact continued to work for, and her fund subsidized, nurse training in workhouse infirmaries to the end of her working life. Moreover, primary sources show that both Mill and Twining were emboldened by contact with Nightingale on the issue; both took stronger positions after than before contact. Dickens's influence came from his novels, and he was never a political reformer. Finally, although Baly acknowledges the work at the Highgate and Marylebone workhouse infirmaries in London, she entirely misses Nightingale's leading role throughout the whole workhouse reform movement.

The Legacy of De-mythologizing

Dingwall, Rafferty, and Webster devote a chapter in *An Introduction to the Social History of Nursing* to "making the myths," which includes nasty remarks about Nightingale's family relations as well as a thorough denunciation of every aspect of her nursing career. The putdowns use sexist language to boot, as in "Florence's cruellest comments."[67] These authors assert that Nightingale's work was not original, and they even misconstrue her advocacy of fundamental system change as mere "personal" philanthropy. They have it backward: "As with other philanthropists, she thought the answer lay in personal work rather than through large-scale social reform."[68] What should one call her advocacy of an entire replacement of the workhouse system with care facilities for the aged, long-term disabled, and chronically ill? Nightingale's "ABCs" of Poor Law reform are no less than a manifesto for fundamental social reform, in effect a proposal for what would be called, after World War II, the welfare state, or social democracy, in much of Europe.

Nightingale's "ABCs of workhouse reform," as she argued them to sanitarian Edwin Chadwick and Poor Law Board president C. P. Villiers, go far beyond the improvement of nursing, significant as that was, to the effective dismantlement of the Poor Law system.

A. To insist on the great principle of separating the sick, insane, infirm and aged, incurable, imbecile, and above all the children from the usual pauper population of the metropolis. (How many of those called incurable are *not* incurable a life's hospital experience has taught me. Old age, is, of course, incurable.)
B. To advocate a single central administration.
C. To place all these classes (especially those suffering from any disease, bodily or mental) under this distinct and responsible administration, amenable directly to Parliament.

These are the ABC's the reform required....Sick, infirm, idiots and mad persons require special constructive arrangements, special medical care and nursing and special dieting. (Of all these, they have little or none that is worthy the name in the present London workhouses.) They are not "paupers." They are "poor and in affliction." Society certainly owes them, if it owes them anything, every necessary care for recovery. In practice, there should be consolidated and uniform administrative arrangements.

Sickness is not *parochial;* it is general and human. For sick you want hospitals as good as the best civil hospitals. You want the best nurses you can find. You want efficient and sufficient medical attendance. You want an energetic and wise administration.[69]

Would the de-mythologizers tell us who had a more profound or radical vision of reform than Nightingale at this time? It would be difficult to find anything of the same scope until the recommendations of the Minority Report on the Poor Law, in 1909, led by Sidney and Beatrice Webb.

As for nursing itself, the de-mythologizers are again incorrect. They deny that Nightingale did any nursing work at her Harley Street establishment, where she did all the organizing of convalescent and posthospital care, as well as the administration, and probably all the admissions: "She was not a deliverer of care but an organizer of others' labour," say Dingwall, Rafferty, and Webster.[70]

As a result of so much focus on "de-mythologizing" Nightingale, a generation of nurses has learned next to nothing about the most illustrious founder of their profession. Depending on where they studied, they may have heard disparaging cracks from witty clinical instructors. That this major founder had a vision of a comprehensive public health-care system, specifying quality care for all, including the poor, in 1864, goes unmentioned. That Nightingale led a team of (male) public health experts, including leading doctors and engineers, to advocate systemic change has not been thought worthy of mention. So also for the fact that she consistently paid attention to occupational health and safety issues for nurses. That her nurses took on the toughest hospital assignments, even the dismal workhouse infirmaries, and went to foreign countries and braved poor conditions there surely might be worth a note.

That Nightingale was a pioneer statistician, responsible for the first comprehensive study of maternal mortality postchildbirth in England, likewise goes unnoted in the nursing world. The statistical analysis she began on her return from the Crimean War would now go by the term "evidence-based health-care."[71] But this, too, has escaped the attention of the de-mythologizers. Her statistical work, however, is recognized in the history of that subject; see, for example, Richard Stone, *Some British Empiricists in the Social Sciences, 1650–1900*.[72] While the de-mythologizers have been so occupied in remaking Nightingale's post-Crimea time as one of psychological and emotional breakdown, they have ignored her massive *Notes on Matters Affecting the Health, Efficiency and Hospital Administration of the British Army*. It was not only ground-breaking statistical analysis at the time, but it laid the foundation for her own decades of work on hospital reform (see chapter 6).

That Nightingale devoted some forty years of her life to improving conditions in India is little known outside specialist circles. This effort began with her getting a comprehensive royal commission established on India—and, like that on the Crimean War, doing much of the background research for it. Nightingale then produced numerous papers on public health in India, rural health promotion, famine prevention and relief, land tenure reform, taxation, municipal self-government, and support for the emerging national independence movement.

There is, moreover, an abundance of primary sources on all these subjects, some scarcely looked at, just waiting for up-and-coming scholars to take on. It is to be hoped that the centenary of Nightingale's death will give impetus to a fresh look at her work as a nursing leader and social reformer, by encouraging researchers to read what she herself wrote, not what the de-mythologizers (in effect, re-mythologizers) have said she did.

THE PASSIONATE STATISTICIAN

M. EILEEN MAGNELLO

On my part this passionate study [of statistics] is not in the least based on a love of science, rather it comes from the fact that I have seen so much of the misery and suffering of humanity, of the irrelevance of laws and Governments.
Letter from Florence Nightingale to Adolphe Quetelet, 12 April 1861

Were I a man of wealth I would see that Florence Nightingale was commemorated, not only by the activities symbolised by the "Lady of the Lamp," but by the activities of the "Passionate Statistician." I would have found a Nightingale Chair of Applied Statistics to carry out the ideals expressed in her letters.
Karl Pearson, The Life, Letters, and Labours of Francis Galton **(1924)**

Florence Nightingale's systematic and groundbreaking use of statistics, along with her development of innovative statistical charts and diagrams, established her distinguished position as a foundational thinker in epidemiology, medical statistics, and outcome research. So exceptional were her statistical talents that she became the first woman to be elected a Fellow to the Statistical Society of London (now the Royal Statistical Society). Yet despite the overwhelming prominence of statistics in her work and life, little is known about her role as the "Passionate Statistician," the sobriquet given to her in 1913 by her first biographer, Sir Edward Cook. Biographers have paid scant attention to the extraordinary role of statistics in Nightingale's work. While many of these scholars include some discussion of statistics in relation to her reports from royal commissions, others comment only that she used statistics in a methodical manner. Her statistical work is often treated as though it were secondary to and quite separate from her ideas about nursing when, it could be argued, the two were often interwoven. Nightingale's extensive use of statistics and her innovative statistical graphs informed her ideas of nursing by providing empirical evidence about the lamentable conditions of nursing. The statistical evidence she accrued enabled her to make many institutional changes, usually with the full support of the government. This chapter traces the path that led to her landmark statistical work in the field of nursing.

The statistical methods and ideas of the Victorian vital statistician William Farr (1807–93) and the Belgian astronomer and social statistician Adolphe Quetelet (1796–1874) provided a conduit for health reforms for the mathematically inclined Florence Nightingale. By using their statistical methods, she persuaded various government officials of the importance of the lessons she learned in the Crimean War and showed that by implementing sanitary reforms in hospitals, mortality rates could be reduced in the army at home. She understood the power of statistics and used them to support her convictions.

Like so many other social and vital statisticians, Nightingale felt empowered by the pervasive passion for statistics that enthralled the Victorians. By the middle of the nineteenth century, Victorian Britain had witnessed an explosion of industrial, technological, and social changes that engendered the coexistence of immense variation and apparent randomness in society. The confluence of these twinned statistical concepts became a source of diversification and quantification that was harnessed by mid-Victorian statisticians to undertake statistical investigations of mass phenomena. This led to a widespread dissemination of statistical information by the middle class through lectures, health tracts, medical advice in the popular press, self-help books, and novels. Charles Dickens's *Hard Times* and George Eliot's *Middlemarch* exemplified how this new statistical language had become a part of the vernacular of the Victorians.

Florence Nightingale was brought up in a liberal-humanitarian household. Her solidly upper-middle-class family were Unitarian dissenters and intellectually adventurous freethinkers (individuals who formed opinions about religion on the basis of reason without recourse

to authority or established beliefs). Her parents were part of the intellectual avant-garde that endorsed women's education.[1] Nightingale's
upbringing thus nourished and stimulated her enthusiasm of mathematics. By the time she was nine years old, she was already organizing
her data in a tabular format and collaborating in a project with male
contemporaries. Her father, a graduate of Trinity College, Cambridge,
included some basic mathematics in her lessons. This edifying background, combined with Nightingale's religious beliefs, played a pivotal
role in shaping her ideas about statistics.

When she was sixteen years old, she recorded that "God had called
her to His service," and she began to study the mystics and comparative
religion. By the time she was in her twenties, she had rejected the super-
natural and miraculous underpinnings of Christianity. To Nightingale,
according to Mark Bostridge, God "was a benevolent being of infinite
goodness and wisdom, wholly unlike the wrathful, punitive deity of
traditional belief."[2] Nightingale thus presented a God with whom man
could enter into partnership, as a "fellow-searcher" after truth.[3] She proposed a form of religion in which human beings actively contributed to
the realization of God's law through their work. Statistical laws provided
her with a viable pathway that could reveal God's providential plan.

In common with the many Victorians who adopted science as the new
religion, she shared the view that the only way to advance science was
by registering facts, utilizing microscopes, and recording and measuring
electrical, mechanical, and physical constants, which were to be applied
to some of the new statistical and mathematical models that were being
developed. Vital statisticians wanted to use these models to improve the
dire situation of the poor and to advocate for public health reforms in the
industrialized cities, where perilous conditions threatened the lives of so
many Victorians.[4]

Nightingale regarded science and statistics as a substitute religion;
statistics was for her "the most important science in the world."[5] Although she took much enjoyment from assembling the dullest and driest
statistical compilations, her writing was, as John Eyler notes, anything
but a dry account of statistics; she wrote with a passionate conviction for sanitary reform.[6] She further maintained that "to understand
God's thought, we must study statistics for these are the measure of His
purpose."[7] She shared with Francis Galton (1822–1911) the idea that "the
statistical study of natural phenomena was the 'religious duty of man.'"[8]
Nightingale's ideology was rooted in the theology of the clergyman

William Derham (1657–1735), from whose ideas she developed her view that "we learn the purpose of God by studying statistics."[9] Moreover, her religious outlook offered her a way to establish the legitimacy of statistics in her work and life. The study of statistics was thus a moral imperative and a religious duty: it was the surest way of learning the divine plan and directing action in accordance with it.

As a young woman, Nightingale met a number of Victorian scientists at dinner parties at the family's winter house in Embley Park, including the mathematician Charles Babbage (1791–1871), who along with Quetelet was one of founders of the Statistical Society of London in 1834. She was so fascinated with numbers at an early age that by the time she was twenty she wanted further tuition in mathematics, and she began receiving two-hour instructions from a tutor, the eminent Cambridge-trained mathematician J. J. Sylvester (1814–97), who later became Savilian Professor of Geometry at Oxford. Her mathematical aptitude fueled her predilection for statistics. In the mornings Nightingale would study material on the statistics of public health and hospitals, and eventually she accumulated a formidable array of statistical information. Her enjoyment was so immense that she found that the sight of a long column of figures was "perfectly reviving." By then she had already read Quetelet's book, whose statistical ideas invigorated her own convictions on the laws of statistics.

Adolphe Quetelet and Statistical Social Laws

Quetelet was one of the primary advocates of adopting natural and astronomical laws and applying them to the body. In the 1830s he was one of the first to use statistical methods to quantify social phenomena by borrowing mathematical tools from astronomers. During this time he popularized the arithmetical mean when he discovered that astronomical error laws (i.e., normal distribution) could be applied to the distribution of human features, such as height and girth. This recognition led, in turn, to his much-celebrated construct, *l'homme moyen* (the average man). Mean values were, however, of scientific value to Quetelet only when they represented a type, as deviations from this average were seen as flawed and a product of error. For Quetelet, the regularities he found in man were comparable with the laws of physics. His realization of the inherent complexity underlying the measurement of social phenomena led him to devise a quantitative system of statistical laws, which he termed "social physics," that ostensibly governed the varying rates of crime, marriage, and suicide. Quetelet borrowed the phrase "social physics" from the French philosopher Auguste Comte (1778–1857), who coined the word "sociology" after he learned that Quetelet had begun using his original term.

Quetelet was convinced that these mean values could be used to find the ideal type of society, politics, and morals. Since he thought that deviations from central values caused society's ills, he believed that a mean philosophical and political position should be able to resolve society's conflicts. His statistical work became a catalyst for a number of social and vital statisticians in mid-Victorian Britain. For Nightingale, Quetelet's ideas of natural statistical laws provided a channel for her intellectual stimulation and a way to understand God's natural phenomena.

Nightingale's parents did not, however, approve of the hours she spent studying mathematics, as she was expected to fulfill her duty by getting married; but she had no interest in the idea of a husband and had rejected the marriage proposal from Richard Monckton Milnes (later Baron Houghton), who became president of the Royal Statistical Society from 1865 to 1867. Much to her parents' consternation, she announced that she wanted to work as a nurse at Salisbury Hospital for several months. She then confessed that she had the idea of eventually setting up a house of her own to establish "something like a Protestant Sisterhood, without vows, for women of educated feeling."[10]

It was the family physician, Sir James Clark, with the support of family friends Sidney and Elizabeth Herbert, who advised Nightingale to leave home and accept an unpaid position as superintendent of a small hospital. By April 1853 she began her work at a hospital she renamed the Institute for Gentlewomen during Illness, at 1 Harley Street, then becoming established as a preeminent area of medicine in London. She even hired the Harley Street physician William Edward Stewart. In her new position Nightingale installed a supply of hot water to all floors and a dumbwaiter to deliver hot food from the kitchen. She then replaced the grocer, the coal merchant, and the kitchen range while reorganizing the bookkeeping and bringing the accounts into order. These early experiences showed her to have a remarkable flair for imposing her will on institutions, as well as an "extraordinarily rich and firm imaginative grasp of the relations between individuals and the sitting and working of things and of human beings' relations to them," as F. B. Smith notes.[11] Nevertheless, Nightingale was suspicious of curative medicine and medical science; her strengths lay, instead, in her administrative and managerial skills with hospitals. Later that year she began to distribute questionnaires on health administration to hospitals in Europe and to record the responses in statistical tables.

A year after Nightingale improved the conditions in the hospital, her lifelong friend and secretary at war, Sidney Herbert, asked her to be "Superintendent of the female nursing establishment in the English General Military Hospitals in Turkey" for the British troops fighting in the Crimean War and to take a group of thirty-eight nurses with her. From her connections with the government and her years of advocacy for professional nursing, she had already gained the prestige that made this exceptional appointment possible. Nightingale and her nurses worked alongside the pensioners and recovering soldiers who traditionally served the sick and wounded during a war. Before this time women had never been allowed to serve officially. Herbert had responded to public outrage at the reports published in *The Times* of the suffering of the common soldier caused by the incompetence of the British army commanders. He hoped Nightingale's presence would pacify the public. Readers of *The Times* donated £7,000 for her personal use, a sum that was eventually used to improve hospital conditions, but it also inspired jealousy among army doctors and officers.

Once Nightingale arrived in the Crimea, she found herself amid utter chaos in the hospital at Scutari: there were no blankets, beds, furniture, food, or cooking utensils, but there were rats and fleas everywhere. She drew the government's attention to matters that went far beyond her sphere of influence and exposed the administrative incompetence and disorganization of the British military. Fortunately, she had an exceptional capacity for large-scale organization and implementation of administrative reform, though she was thought by some to be lacking in patience and the ability to compromise.

Nightingale was dismayed by the statistical carelessness as well as the appalling lack of sanitation she found in the military hospitals. The medical records were in a deplorable state, as none had been maintained in a uniform manner. Moreover, there was a complete lack of coordination among hospitals and no standardized or consistent reporting. Each hospital had its own nomenclature and classification of diseases, which were then tabulated on different forms, making comparisons impossible.

Even the number of deaths was not accurate; hundreds of men had been buried, but their deaths were not recorded. One of the first books Nightingale wrote, *Notes on Matters Affecting Health, Efficiency, and Hospital Administration of the British Army* (1858),[12] which was printed and privately circulated but never published, provided statistical evidence that showed how much of the mortality was due to the conditions of the hospitals. She compared the death rates of the army in peacetime with the civilian rate and concluded that "our soldiers are enlisted to die in barracks." The statistical data Nightingale collected during the first seven months of the Crimean campaign were later analyzed with the help of William Farr.

Nightingale's Statistical Partnership with William Farr

It was Nightingale's close collaborative work with the physician and medically trained statistician William Farr which led to some of her most important statistical work. Farr was one of the foremost vital statisticians in Britain and was sympathetic to her ideas of reforms. When Farr and Nightingale met at a dinner party in the autumn of 1856, he had already initiated the systematic collection and deployment of vital statistics. His work as compiler of abstracts and later as statistical superintendent at the General Register Office (GRO) (now the Office of Population Censuses and Surveys) in 1839 was a landmark in the development of English preventive medicine and medical statistics. Nightingale had just returned from the Crimea a national heroine, albeit an emaciated and tense one. She recognized that if such suffering were never to happen again, the Army Medical Service, and if necessary the army itself, must be reformed. She was about to begin her campaign for reform in the Army Medical Department when they met. They began a correspondence that would continue for twenty years, writing some four hundred letters between them. In November 1856 she requested the formation of a Royal Commission on the Health of the Army, and on her recommendation Farr was appointed a member.

Nightingale gained Farr's expert statistical and actuarial advice along with his support and assistance with most of her statistical reports and papers that she delivered at society meetings. She relied on Farr for the analysis of the army reform returns of death and disease and for some of his tactics of using mortality statistics argumentatively. Due to the nature of his work at the GRO, he had access to unpublished vital statistical records. Farr benefited from Nightingale's politically influential connections and her knowledge about nursing practices in major hospitals. Thus their twinned desires to see reforms in the Army Medical Department led to a fulfilling and productive professional relationship. They also collaborated in the preparation of hospital statistics for her *Notes on Hospitals* (1859) and *Introductory Notes on Lying-in Institutions* (1871).[13] Her *Notes on Hospitals* was popular with general audiences, largely because of its clear, concise style and its practical common sense. Although the first edition (1859) did not contain statistical material, by the third edition, in 1862, a chapter was devoted to statistics.

Nightingale was usually quite demanding in the support she expected from her associates, including many politicians she knew, but she treated Farr with deference and relied on flattery for his cooperation. Eyler suggests that this special treatment had to do with the extraordinary value she attached to statistics; she understood the power statistics had over politicians and how such information could change their firmly established ideas and thus prompt them to implement legal reform.[14]

Given the amount of time Nightingale spent with Farr computing and analyzing death rates, she eventually became quite competent with undertaking this work on her own. When she sent Farr the death rates she computed from her Crimean data in May 1857, he replied, "I have read with much profit your admirable observations. It is like a light shining in a dark place."[15] He was quite enthusiastic about the diagrams and accompanying descriptions he received later that year, letting her know that "your speech is the best that ever was written on diagrams or on the Army."[16]

Analysis of the Crimean data revealed that during the war more troops died from such diseases as typhus, typhoid, and cholera and unsanitary living conditions than in London during the Plague of 1655. Nightingale and Farr discovered there was an annual mortality rate of 60 percent for these soldiers. Between the ages of 25 and 35 the mortality rate in military hospitals was double that in civilian life: whereas 20 per 1,000 died in military hospitals, 10 per 1,000 died in civilian life. The suggestion that the mortality rate of troops in the Crimea was higher than that of the Great Plague may have been due in part to the way Farr calculated hospital mortality.[17]

Nightingale wrote a report based on the army medical statistics and sent it as a confidential communication to the War Office and Army

Medical Department. Farr provided the Army Sanitary Commission with the type of analysis and testimony that Nightingale wanted. Eventually, the army adopted Farr's nosology and classification of disease, with modification. One of the main outcomes of the statistical aspect of the Royal Commission was the creation of a department of Army Medical Statistics. Nightingale and Farr later demonstrated that three times as many soldiers died at home and abroad during peacetime as when they were at war because of overcrowding and filth in the industrialized cities.

Farr was one of the first statisticians to make extensive use of diagrams and other pictorial aids. Like Nightingale, Farr understood that the use of visual aids and graphs should be aimed at those who were not accustomed to looking at statistical data or life tables. He kept this in mind when he wrote up his report on the Army Sanitary Commission. Nightingale developed a flair for devising graphic methods, including her well-known polar area graph, which was similar to the pie chart created by the Scottish economist William Playfair (1759–1823) in 1801. Her polar area graph, which was cut into twelve equal angles, each of which represented one month of the year, revealed changes over time.[18] Her graph not only dramatized the extent of the needless deaths among the soldiers during the Crimean War, but was used as a corrective tool to persuade the medical profession that deaths were preventable if sanitation reforms were implemented. She recognized that when statistical data were made accessible with the use of graphs and charts, they could sway long-held opinions. These statistical illustrations enabled her to demonstrate to government officials that mortality rates could be reduced in the army and in London once sanitary procedures became routine in hospitals. Once Nightingale and Farr had set up their program on army reform, Nightingale turned her attention to the army statistics in India.

Indian Army Statistics

The aftermath of the Indian Mutiny of 1857 gave Nightingale plenty of scope for a new program of statistical analyses in the Indian army. Given the successful statistical work she had been undertaking, she got a Royal Indian Sanitary Commission appointed straightaway, and she was in charge of arranging the staff and managing the project. Farr served on the commission and was paid as an actuarial consultant; he was also given the assistance of four clerks. His official duties involved the collection and analysis of the data. Nightingale sent questionnaires to two hundred stations in India to gather information about troop strength, sickness, and deaths for the previous ten years. Although the commission was issued in May 1859, it was four years before the report was completed; the delay was due to the difficulties in collecting data, with responses often being incomplete or late.

The purpose of Farr's statistical section was to prove that "it is not the climate that sweeps away our soldiers."[19] Since the 1830s Farr had been convinced that the tropics were inherently unhealthy for the English. He had initially blamed lifestyle, climate, or racial differences and not sanitation for the much higher mortality rates among English troops in India than among native Indian troops. Nevertheless, the high mortality of the English troops in India should not have been inevitable. After he analyzed their data, Farr found that he had to reconsider some of his ideas about the "unhealthy tropics": their results indicated that sanitation, and not lifestyle, climate, or racial differences, was the main contributing factor in the high incidence of mortality. He concluded that the English army could indeed live healthily in India. The report recommended reforms in sanitation, barracks and hospital construction, diet and water supply, and discipline, and the formation of a regional sanitary commission.[20] Nightingale was right to stress the fundamental importance of irrigation and the need for a pure water supply. This time spent studying conditions in India conferred considerable political influence on Nightingale. Her knowledge of India became so encyclopedic that every viceroy visited her before leaving Britain.[21]

Hospital Statistics Reforms

In October 1858 Nightingale read a paper on the sanitary conditions of hospitals in London and Scutari at the annual meeting of the National Association for the Promotion of Social Sciences in Liverpool. The findings in the paper led to her book *Hospital Statistics and Hospital Plans* (1862).[22] Her first recommendation was the adoption of the nomenclature of disease used by the Registrar General of England and the use of standardized forms to collect hospital data: the total sick populations (the number of beds in use); the number of cases of diseases receiving medical or surgical treatment, with patients listed by age, sex, and disease; the average stay in the hospital, again broken down by age and sex; and the annual proportion of recoveries by the beds occupied. Farr wanted to have weekly reports in all large cities (based on the London model) in the rest of Europe and in America, too.

Nightingale's investigation of London's hospital statistics confirmed that the recordkeeping in London's hospitals needed to be revised. In addition to just simple carelessness in the collation of statistical information, there was a complete lack of scientific coordination. For example, hospital statistics gave very little useful information on the average duration of hospital treatment or on the proportion of patients who recovered compared with those who died. Likewise, while working as compiler of abstracts to the GRO, Farr had found it deeply troubling that there were so many inconsistencies in the reporting of deaths in English hospitals, which did not use a standard nosology. A Statistical Society Committee was set up for the campaign to keep hospital statistics in a uniform scheme that would permit comparative studies.

Nightingale wanted to establish a standardized form that would list cause of death and create divisions for death by disease, injuries, or following operations. Farr helped advance the project by making her proposals a central topic in the program for the Sanitary Section of the 1860 International Statistical Congress, held in London. It was at this conference that Nightingale met the Belgian statistician Adolphe Quetelet for the first time and argued for the establishment of uniform medical statistics for hospitals. Though her forms were being used in England, she also wanted the standard forms to be adopted throughout Europe, which she hoped would allow comparisons to be made with various European hospitals. The congress endorsed her plan with slight modification and directed that forms and recommendations be sent to all member nations. With this kind of endorsement, she continued to pressure the London hospitals to comply with her forms. The committee on hospital statistics did in fact use the official nosology to report cases enumerated in the London hospitals. Her hospital model forms were printed in 1859 and were adopted in 1861 by St. Bartholomew's, St. Mary's, St. Thomas', University College, and Guy's hospitals; Guy's, which adopted her forms in 1861, advocated that each hospital publish its own statistics annually. Later that year Nightingale issued another popular appeal to the Social Science Association. The results of these hospital reports were published in the *Journal of the Statistical Society of London* in 1862.[23] Though the forms were used for a period of time, the hospitals eventually found them too costly and time-consuming to administer.

Her skills in reporting and illustrating statistical data for sanitary reform and in military and London hospitals eventually brought her official recognition. Nominated by Farr, in October 1858 she was the first woman to be elected a Fellow of the Statistical Society of London, and in the same year she was also elected to the Statistical Congress. She was made an honorary foreign member of the American Statistical Association in 1874.

Her view that the healthiest hospitals were in the provinces while the unhealthy ones were situated in the metropolis of London was based on using mortality as a criterion for assessment rather than hospital infection. Although Nightingale was criticized for her anti-contagion view by Farr and other medical practitioners, she eventually embraced germ theory (today known as the pathogenic theory of medicine), as Lynn McDonald has shown (see chapter 5). Contagionists maintained that diseases arose from bacilli, not from miasma or poisons in the air exuded from rotting animal and vegetable matter, whereas anti-contagionists presumed disease arose from miasma and addressed the problem by trying to make changes in the environment. The germ theory of disease, which showed that microorganisms are the cause of many diseases, led in turn to the development of bacteriology at the end of the nineteenth century. Farr never wavered in his commitment to sanitary reform and accepted the increasing body of new ideas about etiology and pathology.

Later that year Nightingale became involved with the Census of 1861 when she persuaded the GRO to extend its scope by collecting statistics that would serve as a foundation for sanitary reform. She achieved this aim by including a count on Census Day of the sick and infirm, who had not been counted in previous censuses. Though some thought collecting information from invalids would be too cumbersome, Nightingale retorted that it had already been done in Ireland. Her second aim was to obtain complete data on the housing of the population, as had also been done in Ireland. She was convinced, quite rightly, that the relationship between health and housing was important.

Nightingale was also interested in the mortality after operations that stemmed from the prevalence of hospital gangrene and other septic conditions. She wrote a report that Farr suggested she read at the International Statistical Congress held in Berlin in 1863. She had collected data from 482 operations that were fatal due to septic complications and argued that these outcomes were notoriously connected with unsanitary conditions in the wards or with the conditions in some "patients so bad as to render doubtful the propriety of operating."[24]

A Plea for Teaching Statistics

Nightingale had long been aware that although members of Parliament had access to an enormous amount of statistical data, they made no use of this information; their university educations had provided no training about statistical methods. Nightingale thus wanted to establish the teaching of statistics in universities. Since she had already found that an understanding of statistics could save lives, she was convinced that such information would lead others to make appropriate decisions and that government officials, in particular, ought to countenance such a plan. Nightingale argued that ministers legislated without knowing what they were doing, and that the men who were to govern needed to be taught the use of statistical methods in order to understand statistical information.

Lord Brougham, who founded the *Edinburgh Review* and worked as a solicitor in Edinburgh for three years before moving to London in 1803, argued that statistics should be to the legislator what the compass is to the navigator, but the actual course of legislation was often conducted without any such statistical compass. Since cabinet ministers had received no education in statistical methods, Nightingale remarked, the results led to legislation that was "not progressive, but see-saw-y."[25] There were two exceptions to her pithy remarks, her friend and secretary at war, Sidney Herbert, and the bookseller and statesman W. H. Smith (1825–91), who expanded and developed the business his father, William Henry Smith (1792–1865), had started in the Strand in 1820. W. H. Smith served in Parliament from 1868 until his death and held the posts of secretary of the treasury, first Lord of the Admiralty, and first secretary for war.

After Nightingale heard that her esteemed colleague Adolphe Quetelet had died in February 1874, she thought that the best memorial to him would be to introduce his statistics at Oxford. That a Department of Applied Statistics should be established at Oxford was partly due to her association with her old friend Benjamin Jowett (1817–93), a classical scholar and Master of Balliol College who translated the major works of

Plato and Aristotle into English. They first met in 1862, and much of their relationship centered on discussions about religion. Jowett felt considerable affection and devotion toward Nightingale and wanted to help her set up statistical lectures at Oxford.

By New Year's Eve 1876, Jowett had a proposal for endowing a chair of statistics at Oxford. They consulted Francis Galton about the details.[26] He thought, however, that it would be nearly impossible to set up a new professorship at Oxford or Cambridge because the subject was not part of the undergraduate examinations and would inevitably sink into oblivion. Galton was, perhaps, somewhat pessimistic, for in 1891 Oxford appointed the distinguished statistician Francis Ysidro Edgeworth (1845–1926) to the Chair of Political Economy at All Souls College.

Galton suggested instead that it would be more suitable to train applied statisticians by six lectures a year at the Royal Institution. A number of years later the statistician Karl Pearson, and Galton's biographer, remarked that he thought Nightingale had the better scheme because although the "Royal Institution was valuable for announcing in a popular way the results of recent research, it was not an academic center for training enthusiastic young minds to a new department in science."[27] Nonetheless, Pearson thought Nightingale's desire to create such a chair should somehow be commemorated. In 1911, some twenty years after Pearson made this comment, he was looking for a name for his newly established statistics department, and he held that "no fitter and worthy name occurred to me than that of Applied Statistics."[28] But more than a century would pass before Oxford University renamed their Department of Biomathematics the Department of Applied Statistics in 1988.

Nightingale was a practical statistician who showed how statistics could be a powerful tool when used judiciously: her discerning examination of figures informed her that she could save the lives of the wounded and the sick by implementing essential and appropriate sanitary measures. For Nightingale, statistics were a form of currency but of little value if data were simply accumulated and put aside; she thus demonstrated that their real importance lay in the subsequent analysis and interpretation. Hence, the field of statistics was not simply about collecting data or compiling numerical figures; the data had important political and practical value that could lead to parliamentary reform and save lives. By systematizing recordkeeping practices at Scutari, she established that it was essential to ensure that hospital statistics were standardized across all hospitals in London and the rest of the United Kingdom, because this information enabled her to ascertain which diseases were most prevalent in particular hospitals. Moreover, Nightingale's statistical ideas and innovations were deeply interwoven into her religious thinking, which imbued her lifelong goal to reform the practice of nursing. Like many other Victorian scientists and medical practitioners, Nightingale was in the vanguard of the professionalization of medicine, science, and mathematical statistics in the late nineteenth century.

Although Florence Nightingale is rightly acknowledged and highly venerated for her role in reforming nursing in the mid-nineteenth century, she clearly deserves more recognition than she has received for revolutionizing nursing through her use of statistics. She brought about these fundamental changes through her dedication to her many prodigious statistical reports on standardizing hospital statistics and by implementing the use of medical statistics in the nursing profession. This investigative work led to a decline in the many preventable deaths that occurred throughout the nineteenth century in English military and civilian hospitals. Nevertheless, it has to be said that Nightingale's statistical innovations and achievements are as important in the twenty-first century as they were in the mid-nineteenth century. Certainly, making statistical data accessible by using diagrams and charts is imperative for the medical sciences. Moreover, the development of randomized clinical trials in the mid-twentieth century and the growing reliance on evidence-based medicine in the twenty-first century demand an understanding of contemporary statistical methods, which will enable nurses to make informed decisions about current medical research and their patients.

AN ICON AND ICONOCLAST
FOR TODAY

ANNE MARIE RAFFERTY AND ROSEMARY WALL

From Florence Nightingale's School, a stone's throw from St. Thomas' Hospital, we wonder what Miss Nightingale would make of nursing today. Would she applaud its achievements or despair that it had lost its way? The publication of this book in the centenary year of her death and on the one hundred fiftieth anniversary of the Florence Nightingale School of Nursing and Midwifery, direct descendant of the original Nightingale Training School, leads to questions of why we still revere, commemorate, and celebrate Nightingale. To what extent is she a relevant icon for the twenty-first century? Nightingale's skills as a methodologist and communicator in understanding how to pull the levers of power to bring about change are as much in demand today as they ever were. Furthermore, she was a person who challenged authority and long-held assumptions, rejecting practice where it fell short of her beliefs and behaviors. It was this defiance that enabled her to be so successful in her many campaigns and made her the iconoclast she undoubtedly was. Was it this iconoclasm that allowed her to achieve so much and reach so many? How would Nightingale use those skills and knowledge to contribute to current debates to improve patient care and the health of society? What can contemporary nurses learn from this greatest of iconoclasts?

Consider, for example, the influential 2003 report from the United Kingdom National Health Service (NHS), *Modern Matrons: Improving the Patient's Experience,* which recommended a return to the Nightingale idea of a single senior nurse responsible for the overall running of the hospital—nursing care, cleanliness, food quality, and so forth. In fact, the section titled "Matron's 10 Key Responsibilities" could be composed of extracts from Nightingale's *Notes on Nursing.* It's a sad reflection on contemporary health care that the report found it necessary to empha-size the importance of the matron's responsibility to "get the basics right for patients—clean wards, good food, quality care," a role that is claimed to be a new one for nurses, part of a "profound cultural change which puts the patient first." Nightingale would be astonished to read that it has not been obvious that "the key to the matron role is improving the patient experience. That must be central to everything the NHS does. Unless we improve the quality of the patient experience the NHS could end up hitting every target—but missing the point."[1]

Although Nightingale is best known for her work in nursing, it would be more accurate to say she is an icon for health care in general: what Nightingale was interested in was optimal patient care. There is barely a topic or area in the world of health care today to which her writings and teachings do not apply. Perhaps all health-care workers—clinicians, managers, and support staff—should be encouraged to read *Notes on Hospitals.*[2] Sadly, catastrophes of care are not a thing of the past. Good hospital design as a means to enhance the quality of the healing envi-ronment and patient experience is high on the agenda today, and there remains a lot to learn from Nightingale's writings on the subject.[3] It is not only the design of the physical or built environment in which she excelled, but the psychological environment on which she wrote so com-pellingly and with the most exquisite sensitivity and attention to detail. Any reader of *Notes on Nursing* can only marvel at her intelligence, wis-dom, and command of her subject, her exhortations driving her reader toward higher things.[4] Hers is a world in which the moral and the clini-cal were indivisible, and perhaps they should be for us, too. Spurring her probationers to higher standards and thoroughness, she also warned that doing better should not be conflated with thinking better of oneself: higher achievement should be its own reward, and praise should always be tempered with humility.

Nightingale's call for obedience to doctors, albeit loyal not servile obe-dience, may grate on modern ears and need reframing in the context of contemporary health care. Nevertheless, she recognized the importance of teamwork for the effective delivery of health care. She also understood that the smooth running of an organization relies on the work of the many and not the few. She provides the perfect definition of teamwork: "The very essence of all good organisation is, that everybody should do her (or his) own work in such a way as to help and not hinder every one else's work."[5]

Whether we are involved in meeting the WHO's Millennium Development Goals (to end poverty by 2015) or the quality and safety movement, whether the public health and prevention agenda or moving care closer to home, Nightingale speaks to us today. Her very definition of nursing, both sick and health nursing, is highly relevant to modern health care today. She talks of sick and health nursing in a way that has a decidedly contemporary ring to it. "What is nursing? Both kinds of nursing are to put us in the best possible conditions for Nature to restore or to preserve health—to prevent or to cure disease or injury."[6] She is also acutely aware of the power of the environment to shape health outcomes and the need to intervene and change conditions, using a strong evidence base. This emphasis is only likely to increase as the health burden from chronic disease turns into a global epidemic—if, that is, we do not act now.[7] Intervening upstream and changing the social determinants of health is central to sustaining our health systems. Nightingale recognized the urgency and was adept at communicating that sense of pressure and mobilizing opinion to that end. She observed that infant mortality was the most sensitive index of the health of a population and that what we would refer to as health literacy was key to its reduction: "The life duration of babies is the most 'delicate test' of health conditions. What is the proportion of the whole population of cities or country which dies before it is five years old?...The causes of enormous child mortality are perfectly well known...in one word, want of *household* care of health...but how much of this knowledge has been brought into the homes and households and habits of the people, poor or even rich?"[8]

Her solution was to create a cadre of workers known as health missioners and to establish a dual system of nursing—sick and health nursing—to take the maintenance of good health into the home. She regarded district nursing as "'the Star of Bethlehem,' the crown of good nursing and modern civiliser of the poor."[9] Moving care closer to home is now a major plank of health policy, in which community nursing and primary care services have a key role to play, not only managing demand for hospital care but reducing admissions and readmissions, especially for the frail elderly.[10] There is an urgent need to strengthen community nursing services worldwide and retool them for these new roles and demands.

More broadly, Nightingale emphasizes the importance of carrying public health messages and measures into the workplace and schools, what we would call a joined-up approach to policy. Health messaging remains a priority in our health-care systems as part of outreach and expanding access to care. She did not mince her words when criticizing those who were ignorant of sanitary practice or failed to act where they saw neglect. For the primary epidemic, as far as she was concerned, was "folly" rather than disease. To remedy this, she advocated that officials be persuaded through public opinion to drive health in the home to the top of the political agenda. Nightingale's "health-at-home nursing" and its modern-day equivalents are ever more vital with the economic downturn. Her interest in population health was fueled by the modern conviction that, as she put it, "the health of the unity is the health of the community. Unless you have the health of the unity there is no community health."[11]

We can make a strong case for Nightingale as an icon for today and bring countless more examples to bear on the evidence base. Her words speak to us at so many different levels. We continue to struggle with problems that, had we implemented a fraction of what she had fought for, might not be with us today. Take the state of our hospitals. We still battle with excess mortality in hospitals attributable to hospital-acquired infections. Admittedly, such infections have multiple causes, but the organization of care and insistence on strict discipline in implementing hygiene measures are vital to the solution.[12] Illustrative of a global problem, in at least two recent cases in the United Kingdom outbreaks of the deadly *Clostridium difficile* wreaked havoc in hospitals with disastrous consequences for patients, families, and staff. Again, although the cause of the problems was system failure, the description of conditions in wards could have come from the incriminating pen of Nightingale herself.[13]

The tragedy of recent hospital scandals in England is not only that they happened at all but also that nobody stood up to protest and stop what was going on. No one alerted the external authorities to falling standards or the seismic staff cuts. Neither doctors nor nurses took a stand on the chaos that reigned in some parts of the hospital. The complaints from patients and their families, the neglect experienced by some patients, the tasks left undone, the unanswered call bells, the uneaten food, the patients left lying in soiled sheets for hours on end at risk of pressure sores all went unheeded. The catastrophe is one of the failure of moral courage to take a stand and to accept personal responsibility as professionals. Yet it would not need the intellectual prowess of Florence Nightingale to know what was going wrong. The report by the Health-care Commission (2009), the regulatory watchdog for health care and public health in England and Wales, highlighted deficiencies in the running of the organization at every level. Data on excess mortality were explained away and attributed to coding errors, no follow-up was put in place to secure remedial action, savage cuts in nursing and medical staff were made to meet financial targets, and a catalog of patient complaints about poor nursing care was left to languish.[14] Such problems are clearly not confined to the United Kingdom. In the United States, too, scandal (and major political fallout) arose out the *Washington Post*'s revelations in 2007 of the shocking conditions of veterans at the Walter Reed Military Hospital in Washington, D.C. There investigators found vermin, mold, and sections without heat or water.[15] Charges of staff training failures and administrative incompetence in such instances are reminiscent of what Nightingale found in the Crimea. She spent her life trying to improve the conditions in military hospitals. It is clear that those lessons can be a point of reference today.

Taking our lead from Nightingale, we need to integrate nurses into designing health systems and to recognize this role as an essential driving force of innovation in patient care. One step in the right direction is England's Productive Ward Series, an innovative scheme that provides nurses and other care providers with release time in order to improve patient safety and efficiency.[16] The ability to redesign processes and to work together to improve patient care is precisely what Nightingale exemplified so well and nurses have a prerogative to ensure. She recognized that nurses have the closest and most frequent contact with patients and provide the surveillance system so crucial for overseeing and monitoring care: the "medical man sees the patient only once a day or twice a week"; nurses, observing patients all day every day, can detect and record the subtle changes. If nurses became as vigilant as Nightingale recommends, "it is quite incalculable the good that would certainly come from such sound and close observation in this almost neglected branch of nursing, or the help it would give the medical man."[17] The monitoring and continuous improvement of care is also a key lever in driving up the quality of care. It will enable high-quality recruits to be attracted in an

increasingly competitive labor market, as well as provide the best preparation for practice in modern complex health care. Although including nurses in the redesign of health systems would inevitably involve
costs, it would also bring cost savings in the form of lower morbidity and
mortality and better outcomes for patients. Despite the impressive start
Nightingale made in providing a research base for nursing interventions
and health outcomes, progress has been remarkably slow, and hospital
scandals have not been consigned to the distant past.

To make the contrary case, we might argue, however, that Nightingale is no longer an icon, or is one who has lost her influence, for
had she been so, surely the cases we discuss above would not have occurred. Had staff members been equipped with the skills she possessed
they would have spotted the sentinel signs of chaos within hours: the
undersupply of equipment, the understaffing of units, inadequate in-
vestment in staff training, and an inappropriate skills mix mismatched
to patient acuity. They would have scrutinized the mortality statistics,
looked at the trend data, and taken immediate action. They would have
been impatient with the oversight regime provided by external authorities. They would have insisted that every organization have an early
warning system that was simple to use and demonstrated when standards were deteriorating. They would have driven through change and
not drowned in bureaucratic detail and a morass of metrics. Parsimony
would have been the principle of measurement and coordination of effort. They would have provided leadership to staff, instilling in them a
strong sense of personal responsibility, discipline, and thoroughness in
everything they did.

So perhaps the fact that we still struggle with many of the same challenges as in Nightingale's day points to the limitations of the icon's appeal and influence. Indeed, we might argue that what we need today is
less of the icon and more of the iconoclast. Nightingale may have been
an icon in her own day, but it was her iconoclasm that enabled her to
tear down the barriers that kept so many women captive to social convention. That iconoclasm helped her break free of the stifling world of
enforced female idleness and make her way in a masculine world. It is
that same iconoclasm, moral outrage, and courage to challenge systems,
administrators, or colleagues in cases of professional incompetence, system failure, or unsafe care that we need today.

It is easy as a profession to stand back and throw our hands up in horror at the all-too-frequent high-profile scandals in which our health-care

systems are shown to be dangerous to those in our care, but what are we going to do to take the lessons forward and ensure that such mistakes do not happen again? Are we prepared to do what Nightingale would have done, take responsibility for our actions, act as the sentinel forces for change, raise the alarm and mobilize for that change? We have the evidence base from which to operate and leverage change.[18] We have policies in place to enable us to measure and manage quality of care effectively.[19] We have the ingredients to make change happen, but magnificent metrics and shiny information technology systems are for naught if we do not have the leadership, accountability, and authority to lead the charge and put the data to work to bring about change, drive up standards, and root out poor performance. Patients and their families want good care all the time, not just some of the time. They also want to be treated as individuals and to have continuity in the system.[20]

So what has gone wrong? How have we lost our way? What has happened to leadership in recent times? One answer is that roles have been stretched in too many directions. Combining nursing with other functions such as operations, quality, or human resources has taken our eye off the target. While some have found this attractive as a platform for influence, the role of nursing at the board level and the vesting of authority and accountability in the nurse director has been diluted by other organizational functions.[21] It has taken the focus of attention away from the fundamentals of nursing care and set these up in competition with other concerns, spreading the nurse executive function too thinly. There is a strong case for revisiting the Nightingale notion of vesting authority and accountability for nursing in one head. The public would welcome it.[22]

We need to refocus leadership on the things that matter to patients not just at the top but throughout the entire organization and system. The role of the ward sister/manager in particular needs to be strengthened.[23] It is here that Nightingale is the most convincing, and we can turn to her for inspiration. Her words sparkle on the page with their simple beauty and work their magic on the mind. *Notes on Nursing* provides the perfect tutorial in how to make the patient comfortable, provide a healing environment, and allay the anxieties that may attend the care of the sick, in this case in the home. What it also shows is that Nightingale's skill and dexterity in this domain was of a high order—the many thoughtful touches are indicative of someone who used her intelligence and formidable powers of communication to demonstrate how much of the quality of care is contained in the detail.[24]

In her letter to the nurses and probationers trained under the Nightingale Fund in London in 1897, Nightingale reminded her audience that "nursing is in general made up of little things; little things they are called, but they culminate in matters of life or death."[25] How true this is: it is the detail that gets lost in the clamor to do more and do it faster in the ever-quickening pace of health care. The result is that some patients leave our hospitals worse off than when they entered. In extreme cases they die of malnutrition, develop pressure sores, suffer untreated pain, or develop life-threatening complications. Her clarion cry—"it may seem a strange principle to enunciate as the very first requirement in a Hospital that it should do the sick no harm"—rings in our ears.[26] We call ourselves a caring, even *the* caring, profession, but how can we be discharging our duty when patients are neglected, suffer needlessly, and are left to fend for themselves? It is time to follow Nightingale's lead and take a hard and honest look at ourselves, examine our collective conscience, reflect on where we have been and where we are heading before resetting the compass.

Again we can turn to Nightingale to help us on our way. Nightingale was adamant that those who entered nursing should do so for the right motives. She was obsessed with the higher nature of the calling, and her letters to probationers are filled with spurs to strive for higher standards. But she was equally convinced that at no time should nursing be conducted for the sake of the nurse. Striving to do better should be its own reward. The greatest sin in a nurse was conceit: "if you wish to do what you like and what you do well for the sake of being praised by others, then you nurse for your own vanity, not for the sake of Nursing. But if you wish to be trained to do all Nursing well, even what you do not like—trained to perfection in little things—that is Nursing for the sake of Nursing: for the sake of God and of your neighbour. And remember, in little things as in great, No Cross, no Crown."[27]

Nightingale was conscious of the need to keep her own motives in check. She stressed the importance of humility and was wary of the temptations that reputation and renown could bring in its wake. Perhaps for our part too as a profession we have been motivated by the wrong reasons, seduced by higher rewards that give us more power and prestige but have caused us to lose sight of what patients really want. Perhaps we have been worshiping the false gods of finance and power in some cases and have turned into Pharisees, as Nightingale feared. Perhaps now is the time to smash the icons and make a fresh start. Who or what, then, should be our guiding star?

It was standards and thoroughness in the fundamentals of care that Nightingale insisted on and cherished above all else: the nurse must be

> thorough and perfect in every detail of Ward work, of order and cleanliness, and down to the temperature of a hot water bottle...of a poultice. The smallest thing is important to a Patient, to that most delicate instrument, the human body. We are justly horrified at a mistake in giving medicine or stimulant. We are not perhaps so horrified as we should be at mistakes in fresh air, feeding helpless Patients, cleanliness, warmth, order, and all the rest of what we are taught that Nursing helps Nature and the Physician and Surgeon. It is straightness that is so much wanted; straightness of purpose, work, conduct.[28]

These standards for nurses outlined by Nightingale need to be underpinned by values, and we must ensure that we recruit to those values, behaviors, and capabilities that make up the portrait of the excellent nurse. Nightingale rejected the notion of profession in her day, believing it debased nursing as a calling, undermined the esprit de corps so vital for maintaining the moral tone of practice, and stereotyped mediocrity. She was suspicious of book-learning for its own sake, especially if divorced from apprenticeship. Training, in her view, needed to be multifaceted—"all that, in fact, goes to the full development of our faculties, moral, physical and spiritual." It could be perfected only by the blend of books, apprenticeship on the wards, and supervision, being checked by a sister. One of the "dangers" she identified was basing training on book-learning and lectures rather than an apprenticeship, a workshop practice.[29] In our own time we must strive for the highest standards in training and education to match those of practice. In today's parlance that means degree-based entry into the profession. An education that trains all the faculties in harmony with one another needs to be based in a university setting, for it is here that epidemiology, statistics, social and behavioral science, ethics, law, and the arts can be learned.

It was Nightingale's attentiveness to what we would call the evidence base which was a hallmark of her own practice, specifically statistics as an instrument for informing policy and as a vital part of the government process. These skills are required for not only policymakers but all who are engaged in decision making at the clinical level. All nurses need to be data literate and have the capability to use and interpret data appropriately. Some elements of the skill set were exemplified by Nightingale, and we should define these for different levels of education as core elements of the "Nightingale" curriculum. Her passion for measurement, rigor, and the discipline and dynamics of data are ever more in demand today in a health-care world that measures outcomes, sets benchmarks, and manages performance. The current focus on measurement is certainly one that Nightingale would welcome. Ensuring that nurses have the skills and confidence to appraise and critique the quality of evidence, interpret its significance, and present and communicate it should be part of the educational preparation of every professional nurse. A basic grounding in epidemiological methods, social and behavioral sciences, statistics, evidence-based decision making, policy, and political science as well as the basic and clinical sciences should be part of the "mental equipment" of every nurse, as provided in a degree-based education. Only such an education can confer the confidence that nurses need to stand up for standards and challenge poor practice and conditions that compromise the quality of care. Standards, standards, standards should be our battle cry.

The mechanisms to maintain health and prevent disease are very much in the forefront of current health policy, and with today's economic conditions they are likely to grow in prominence. The need to intervene upstream and prevent the development of avoidable conditions, especially those mediated by behavior and lifestyle, is consistent with Nightingale's teaching and precepts on health nursing.[30] Today it is advocated that care be delivered closer to home, but home was the locus of care in Nightingale's day. The vital contribution of prevention to health and the development of health nursing have almost certainly fallen well short of the progress Nightingale envisioned. Military health remains a major issue, although warfare is very different now and the nature of modern combat brings different health challenges in its wake.

Nightingale both inspired and polarized audiences. There is Nightingale the first-class methodologist, exquisite communicator, politically astute puller of levers, but there is also the petulant Nightingale, scheming and calculating. Then there is the warm, generous, funny, flirtatious Florence, a dear friend and fiendish foe. She had a talent for intimacy, getting the best out of people and drawing people into her world. When her light shone on an individual, it must have felt radiant, intoxicating. She used every scrap of talent, molecule of energy, and resource she had at her disposal to further her ends and objectives. She probably never felt off duty: the clock was ticking, and she might die before her work was done. It was not just what she did but how she did it: her skill was as much a triumph of style as it was of substance. It is her flaws, which make her human and vulnerable, as well as her titanic talents that make her fascinating. Even as we are brought closer to understanding Florence Nightingale's own quest as a "Searcher after Truth," will we ever succeed in our quest as a searcher after the truth about Miss Nightingale? She will continue to enthrall millions who tread in her path.

At the Nightingale School today, no less than in the past, we are intent on ensuring that our students learn the clinical subjects and skills that Nightingale believed were the components of competence. It is the character and comportment of the nurse that underpins the sense of professional responsibility to accept accountability for care and exercise the leadership to stand up for standards, as vital today as it was in Nightingale's reform efforts. Although Nightingale was from a privileged background and drew self-confidence and assurance from being a member of the elite, we need to instill that same self-confidence in our staff and students, nurturing their capability to articulate care through education and the development of their leadership skills.

We need Nightingales for the twenty-first century providing the moral and scientific leadership necessary to advocate for patients using best evidence to deliver effective, safe and compassionate care. The words of Nightingale ring true for us today. The continuous need to improve the quality of health-care is a constant quest of all health systems but that quest comes first and foremost from the individual.

Nightingale was an icon in her own day and as much an icon for health care today, but she left a complex legacy. Are there aspects of Nightingale that are off-putting to upcoming generations of would-be nurses? Is her image one that continues to inspire? Has her iconic status cast a long shadow over others who came in her wake, eclipsing them from view? Our reliance on such a giant has its downside, and history has not elevated her contemporaries or others who walked in her footsteps. Perhaps it is time to take a fresh look at history as well as ourselves as a profession. We need to seek out other heroines not only of the Crimea but in our everyday practice, those who fulfill the Nightingale mission unsung but steadfast in their path. We can ask whether our reliance on Nightingale as such a towering iconic figure is a hindrance to our goal of establishing a diverse talent base for the future. She was a member of the elite, yet the profession molded in her image does not reflect patrician privilege. Perhaps we should cleave a fresh path in which nurses find their inner iconoclast as the standard bearers of a new professionalism—measuring, benchmarking performance in evidence-informed ways, leading innovation in care design and delivery, challenging unacceptable variations in standards of care, valuing interdependence as much as independence, and forming a coalition with patients, the public, and other professionals in mobilizing for change. In doing so we need to be mindful of the lessons of history and of creating a legacy of which Nightingale herself would be truly proud. Nightingale provides the perfect exemplar of the icon, both like and magically unlike ourselves.[31]

NOTES

Introduction

1. E. T. Cook, *Life of Florence Nightingale*, 2 vols. (London: Macmillan, 1913), remains a major text. Among recent biographies is Mark Bostridge, *Florence Nightingale: The Making of an Icon* (New York: Macmillan, 2008).

2. Christopher Hamlin, *Public Health and Social Justice in the Age of Chadwick: Britain, 1800–1854* (Cambridge: Cambridge University Press, 1998).

3. Florence Nightingale, *Notes on Nursing: What It Is and What It Is Not* (1859; New York: Appleton, 1860).

4. Monica Baly, *Florence Nightingale and the Nursing Legacy* (1986; London: Whurr, 1997), 42.

5. "Death of Miss Florence Nightingale," *Guardian*, 15 August 1910, http://century.guardian.co.uk/1910-1919/Story/0,126410,00.html.

6. Susan Reverby, *Ordered to Care: The Dilemma of American Nursing, 1850–1945* (Cambridge: Cambridge University Press, 1987).

7. Nightingale, *Notes on Nursing*.

1. The Nightingale Imperative

1. The Nightingale Pledge was written in Illinois in 1893 by Lystra Gretter, an instructor of nursing at the old Harper Hospital in Detroit, Michigan. "Nightingale Pledge, a Statement of Principles for the Nursing Profession, Formulated by a Committee in 1893," American Nurses Association, http://www.nursingworld.org/FunctionalMenuCategories/AboutANA/WhereWeComeFrom_1/FlorenceNightingalePledge.aspx.

2. Ryoko O'Hara, "An Oral History of Nurses Who Cared for the Atomic Bomb Victims in Hiroshima from August 1945 to the End of That Year" (Ph.D. dissertation, University of Sydney, 2008), xx.

3. Margaret MacMillan, *The Uses and Abuses of History* (London: Profile Books, 2008), 187.

4. John Fortier, "George W. Bush and Truman Parallels Have Abounded," The Hills, http://thehill.com/john-fortier/bush-truman-parallels-2007-05-30.html

5. MacMillan, *Use and Abuses of History*, 100.

6. Ibid., 75.

7. Sioban Nelson, *Say Little, Do Much: Nursing, Nuns, and Hospitals in the Nineteenth Century* (Philadelphia: University of Pennsylvania Press, 2001), 72–75.

8. Judith Godden has written the biography of the Nightingale nurse Lucy Osburn, who brought the model to Australia; see *Lucy Osburn, a Lady Displaced: Florence Nightingale's Envoy to Australia* (Sydney: Sydney University Press, 2006).For the role of Nightingale in the modernization movement in France, see Katrin Schultheiss, *Bodies and Souls: Politics and the Professionalization of Nursing in France, 1880–1922* (Cambridge, Mass.: Harvard University Press, 2001). On Japan, see Aya Takahashi, *The Development of the Japanese Nursing Profession* (London: Routledge 2004). On Brazil, see Ieda de Alencar Barrera, "The Beginnings of Nursing in Brazil: Brazilian Sanitarians and American Nurses," *Nursing History Review* 10 (2002): 33–47.

9. J. M. MacKenzie, *Propaganda and Empire: The Manipulation of British Public Opinion* (Manchester: Manchester University Press, 1984).

10. Florence Nightingale to Henry Parkes, 24 October 1866. *Copy Correspondence between Colonial Government and Florence Nightingale and Others with Reference to the Introduction of Trained Nurses for the Sydney Infirmary and Dispensary* (Sydney: Joseph Cook, 1867), 50.

11. See Godden, *Lucy Osburn*, for a full account; see also chapter 3.

12. Sioban Nelson, "Hairdressing and Nursing: Presentation of Self and Professional Formation in Colonial Australia," *Collegian* 8, no. 2 (2001): 28–31.

13. Lucy Osburn to Florence Nightingale, 24 March 1870, British Library Additional Manuscripts (hereafter BL Add. Mss) 47757 ff 113–18, Mitchell Library, Sydney, Australia.

14. Nelson, *Say Little, Do Much*, 93–94.

15. Katie Pickles, *Transnational Outrage: The Death and Commemoration of Edith Cavell* (Basingstoke, U.K.: Palgrave Macmillan, 2007), 165; and Pickles, *Female Imperialism and National Identity* (Manchester: Manchester University Press, 2002).

16. Pickles, *Transnational Outrage*, 95.

17. Ibid., 165.

18. Freda McDonnell, *Miss Nightingale's Young Ladies: The Story of Lucy Osburn and Sydney Hospital* (Sydney: Angus and Robertson, 1970), 31.

19. Ministry of Health Singapore, *More Than a Calling: Nursing in Singapore since 1885* (Singapore: Grace Communications, 1997), 5.

20. Ann McGrath, "White Brides: Images of Marriage across Colonizing Boundaries," *Frontiers* 23, no. 3 (2002): 76–108; Ann Laura Stoler, "Sexual Affronts and Racial Frontiers: European Identities and Cultural Politics of Exclusion in Colonial Southeast Asia," in *Tensions of Empire: Colonial Cultures in a Bourgeois World*, ed. Frederick Cooper and Ann Laura Stoler (Berkeley: University of California Press, 1997), 198–237.

21. Lucy Osburn to Florence Nightingale, 24 March 1870, BL Add. Mss 47757 ff 127–32, Mitchell Library, Sydney, Australia.

22. Anne Marie Rafferty and Diana Solano, "The Rise and Demise of the Colonial Nursing Service: British Nurses in the Colonies, 1896–1966." *Nursing History Review* 15 (2007): 147–54.

23. Benedict Anderson, *Imagined Communities: Reflections on the Origins and Spread of Nationalism*, rev. ed. (London: Verso, 1991), 6.

24. Barbara Brush and Joan Lynaugh, eds., *Nurses of All Nations: A History of the International Council of Nurses, 1899–1999* (Philadelphia: Lippincott, 1999).

25. Lucien Lefebre, "Combat pour l'histoire," cited in A. Jones, "Word and Deed: Why a Post-structural History Is Needed and How It Might Look," *Historical Journal* 43, no. 2 (2000): 533.

26. "Nightingale Bricks," *British Journal of Nursing* 80 (1932): 203.

27. Royal Melbourne Hospital, "A Nightingale Brick in Australia," *British Journal of Nursing* 85 (1937): 6.

28. "Gifts of Nightingale Bricks," *British Journal of Nursing* 85 (1937): 224.

29. Heide Miller, "Registering the History of Nursing," *Image: Journal of Nursing Scholarship* 24, no. 3 (1992): 241–45.

30. Ibid., 244.

31. Mary Breckinridge, *Wide Neighborhoods: A Story of the Frontier Nursing Service* (1952; Lexington: University Press of Kentucky, 1981), 152.

32. Eric Hobsbawm and Terence Ranger, *The Invention of Tradition* (Cambridge: Cambridge University Press, 1983), 2.

33. Patricia Benner, *Novice to Expert: Excellence and Power in Clinical Nursing Practice* (Menlo Park, Calif.: Addison-Wesley, 1984).

34. Pierre Bourdieu, *The Logic of Practice*, trans. R. Nice (Cambridge: Polity Press, 1990).

35. Michel Foucault, "Technologies of the Self," in *Technologies of the Self: A Seminar with Michel Foucault*, ed. L. H. Martin, H. Gutma, and P. H. Hutton (London: Tavistock, 1988), 16–49.

36. Nightingale Pledge, American Nurses Association.

37. See Minette Marrin "Oh Nurse, Your Degree Is a Symptom of Equality Disease," *Sunday Times* 17 November 2009; or Jessica Shepherd, "Keeping Nursing Students on Course," *The Guardian*, 24 November 2009, for a sample of the debate.

38. International Council of Nurses, "About Us," http://www.icn.ch/abouticn.htm

39. Penny Summerfield, *Reconstructing Women's Wartime Lives: Discourse and Subjectivity in Oral Histories of the Second World War* (Manchester: Manchester University Press, 1998), xiii, 338; Maurice Halbwach, *On Collective Memory* (Chicago: University of Chicago Press, 1992).

40. Ernest Gellner, *Thought and Change* (Chicago: University of Chicago Press, 1964), 169.

41. Mangan J. A., ed., *Imperial Curriculum: Racial Images and Education in the British Colonial Experience* (New York: Routledge, 1993).

42. Bill Ashcroft, *Post-colonial Transformations* (London: Routledge, 2001), 37.

43. M. I. Padhila and S. Nelson, "Teaching Nursing History," *Nursing Inquiry*, Special History Issue, 16 (June 2009): 171–80.

44. M. I. Padhila and S. Nelson, "Networks of Identity: The Potential of Biographical Studies for Teaching Nursing History," *Nursing History Review* (forthcoming).

45. Unison, http://www.unison.org.uk/.

46. http://www.nighcommunities.org/.

47. Deva-Marie Beck, Nightingale Initiative for Global Health, http://www.nighcommunities.org/prayer/.

48. http://www.nighcommunities.org/nighinitiative/.

49. K. K. Hisami, "Florence Nightingale's Influence on the Development and Professionalization of Nursing in Japan," *Nursing Outlook* 44, no. 66 (1996): 284–88; Carol Helmstadter, "Early Nursing Reform in Nineteenth-century London: A Doctor-Driven Phenomenon," *Medical History* 46, no. 3 (2002): 325–50.

50. Sioban Nelson, "From Salvation to Civics: Service to the Sick in Nursing Discourse," *Social Science and Medicine* 53, no. 9 (2001): 1217–25.

2. Navigating the Political Straits in the Crimean War

1. During the Crimean War (1854–56) the English and French armies fought mostly on Russian territory, in the Crimea, but Nightingale herself actually spent more time in the Scutari hospitals in Turkey than she did in the Crimean hospitals. Contemporaries

usually referred to the war theater as "the East" because the war had begun in the Danubian principalities of Moldavia and Wallachia and was fought in the Baltic, the Caucasus, and the Far East as well.

2. Richard W. Davis, *Dissent in Politics, 1780–1830: The Political Life of William Smith, MP* (London: Epworth, 1971), xiii–xv, 250; Barbara Montgomery Dossey, *Florence Nightingale: Mystic, Visionary, Healer* (Springhouse, Pa.: Springhouse Corp., 1999), 24–26, 31–32.

3. Dossey, *Florence Nightingale*, 26.

4. Florence Nightingale (hereafter FN) to her father, 30 August 1853, Wellcome Trust, London (hereafter Wellcome), Ms 8994/38; FN [to Parthenope], 30 September 1853, Wellcome Ms 8994/44. FN to her father, 3 December 1853, British Library Additional Manuscripts (hereafter BL Add. Mss) 45790 ff 152–56.

5. Lord Stanmore, *Sidney Herbert, Lord Herbert of Lea: A Memoir*, 2 vols. (London: John Murray, 1906), 1:332–36.

6. Sir Edward Cook, *The Life of Florence Nightingale*, 2 vols. (London: Macmillan, 1913), 1:146–50; FN to Sidney Herbert, 25 December 1854, BL Add. Mss 43393 ff 45–50.

7. Mother Francis Bridgeman, "An Account of the Mission of the Sisters of Mercy in the Military Hospitals of the East," in *The Crimean Journals of the Sisters of Mercy 1854–56*, ed. Maria Luddy (Dublin: Four Courts Press, 2004), 123–24. Evidence of the Duke of Newcastle, Parliamentary Papers 1854–55, Vol. IX: 132.

8. In practice, Protestants such as William Smith, a Dissenter, did hold office, either by ignoring the rule that they had to receive Communion in the Anglican rite or by "occasional conformity," receiving such Communion once a year. Roman Catholics were not prepared to do this. In the eighteenth century an annual indemnity act was usually passed once a year for persons serving in municipal corporations.

9. "Dissent" and "Nonconformity" were the names given to those Protestant denominations that were not Anglican.

10. Davis, *Dissent in Politics*, xiii, 217–18, 248; Owen Chadwick, *The Victorian Church*, 2 vols. (London: Adam & Charles Black, 1966), 1:2–6; D. G. Paz, *Popular Anti-Catholicism in Mid-Victorian England* (Stanford, Calif.: Stanford University Press, 1992), 1–3.

11. FN, Draft Rules, [1853], Wellcome Ms 8994/89; Mark Bostridge, *Florence Nightingale: The Making of an Icon* (New York: Farrar, Straus & Giroux, 2008), 189.

12. K. Theodore Hoppen, *The Mid-Victorian Generation, 1846–1886* (Oxford: Oxford University Press, 1998), 559.

13. F. K. Prochaska, *Women and Philanthropy in Nineteenth Century England* (Oxford: Faber, 1980), 1–5, citation on 4.

14. FN [to Selina Bracebridge], [c. 15 October 1854], Wellcome Ms 8994/113 ff 1–2, citation on f 1; FN to Elizabeth Herbert, 14 October 1854, BL Add. Mss 43396 ff 10–13.

15. FN to Mary Mohl, 4 May 1853, BL Add. Mss 43397 ff 308–09; FN to Elizabeth Herbert, 14 October 1854, BL Add. Mss 43396 ff 10–13.

16. Selina Bracebridge to "My dearest Mary," October [1854], Nightingale Collection 2/3/B1, Boston University Nursing Archives.

17. For a more detailed discussion of the status of nursing in the 1850s, see Carol Helmstadter, "Shifting Boundaries: Religion, Medicine, Nursing and Domestic Service in Mid-Nineteenth Century Britain," *Nursing Inquiry* 16, no. 2 (2009): 133–43.

18. Nurses Sent to Military Hospitals in the East (hereafter Nurses Sent), [1856], Florence Nightingale Museum, London (hereafter FNM), H01/ST/NC/8/1. The two minor aristocrats were the Honorable Harriet Erskine, a Park Village sister, and Jane Shaw Stewart, who came out in Mary Stanley's party. Victor Bonham-Carter, ed., *Surgeon in the Crimea: The Experiences of George Lawson, Recorded in Letters to His Family, 1854–55* (London: Constable, 1968), 164; Thomas Jay Williams, *The Park Village Sisterhood* (London: SPCK, 1965), 91, 100.

19. Bermondsey Annals, 1854:219, 1855:252–53, citation on 252–53, Archives of the Convent of Mercy, London. See also Helmstadter, "Shifting Boundaries," 135–36.

20. Cook, *Florence Nightingale*, 1:151–54, citations on 153.

21. Roberts was an assistant nurse at St. Thomas' Hospital from 1829 to 1840 and sister of a surgical ward from 1840 to 1853. Nightingale considered her the best of the hospital nurses in the East. Matron's Ward Register, London Metropolitan Archives (hereafter LMA), H01/ST/C2/1, no pagination; Cash Book 1852–58, ST/D7/21, 150; John Flint South, *Facts Relating to Hospital Nurses* (London: Richardson Brothers, 1857), 14–15.

22. FN to Henry Bonham-Carter, 20 December 1892, BL Add. Mss 47724 ff 194–97, citation on f 195; I. B. O'Malley, *Florence Nightingale, 1820–1856* (London: Thornton Butterworth, 1934), 344; FN Note c. 1867, BL Add. Mss 47715 f 23; FN Note, 2 March 1859, Wellcome Ms 7204/Part 2/1 f 4.

23. FN to Herbert, 16 October 1854, Herbert Papers, Wiltshire County Record Office, Chippenham, U.K., 2057/F4/66; Cook, *Florence Nightingale,* 1:155–57; FN to Sir John Hall, 15 October 1855, BL Add. Mss 39867 ff 44–46.

24. Cook, *Florence Nightingale,* 1:158–60; Carol Helmstadter, "Robert Bentley Todd and the Origins of the Modern Trained Nurse," *Bulletin of the History of Medicine* 67 (1993): 297–302. Three Fry nurses went to the army hospitals, and three to the naval hospital at Therapia in 1855. Nurses Sent, 17–18, FNM/H01/ST/NC8/1; Minutes of Committee, 20 October 1854, Wellcome Ms SA/QNI/W2/4. FN to Mother Lydia Sellon, 5 March 1855, Nightingale Collection, Pusey House, Oxford; FN to Lord Panmure, 5 March 1855, WO 43/963, National Archives, U.K. The Victorians called her team secular rather than using the modern term "interdenominational." By secular they meant nondenominational rather than the modern meaning of nonreligious. Sioban Nelson, *Say Little, Do Much: Nurses, Nuns, and Hospitals in the Nineteenth Century* (Philadelphia: University of Pennsylvania Press, 2001), 5.

25. Bishop Thomas Grant to Mother Mary Clare Moore, 20 October 1854, and Moore to Sister Mary Aloysius, 22 October 1854, Bermondsey Annals, 1854:218–19, 222–23, citations on 218 and 223. Cook, *Florence Nightingale,* 1:158–59, 162; Nurses Sent, [1856], FNM/ST/H01/NC8/1.

26. FN [to Selina Bracebridge,] [c. 15 October 1854], Wellcome Ms 8994/113 ff 1–2, citation on f 2.

27. Five were in Turkey: the Barrack and the General hospitals were in Scutari; the Upper and the Lower hospitals were in Koulali; and the Palace Hospital for officers. In the Crimea there were four: the Balaclava General, the Castle, the Land Transport, and the Monastery hospitals. There was a convalescent hospital at Abydos, 125 miles from Scutari, and there were four hulks anchored off Scutari which accommodated one thousand patients. Convalescents were also sent to Malta and Corfu. John Shepherd, *The Crimean Doctors: A History of the British Medical Services in the Crimean War,* 2 vols. (Liverpool: Liverpool University Press, 1991), 1:175–76, 2:343. With the exception of the Monastery Hospital in the Crimea, the government-paid nurses were not employed in the convalescent hospitals. In addition, there were two civil (or civilian) hospitals, one in Smyrna and one in Renkioi, in which government-paid nurses worked. Nightingale was not responsible for those nurses, but when the hospitals closed, she took a number of them into the military hospitals. These hospitals were called civil because they were staffed by civilian, not army, doctors. John Shepherd, "The Civil Hospitals in the Crimea (1855–56)," *Proceedings of the Royal Society of Medicine* 59, no. 3 (1966): 199–204.

28. FN to Herbert, 15 December 1854, BL Add. Mss 43393 ff 34–40.

29. FN to her family, [29 November 1849], Wellcome Ms 9018/7; FN to her family, [December 1849], Wellcome Ms 9018/8, citation on f 10; FN to Harry Bonham-Carter, 9 August 1867, BL Add. Mss 47715 ff 12–13.

30. For example, see Bostridge, *Florence Nightingale,* 291, or FN to Uncle Sam Smith, 6 March 1856, BL Add. Mss 45792 ff 17–18.

31. Bermondsey Annals, 1854:227–28; Cook, *Florence Nightingale,* 1:182–83.

32. Carol Helmstadter, "Early Nursing Reform in Nineteenth Century London: A Doctor-Driven Phenomenon," *Medical History* 46 (2002): 328–33; Memorandum of Agreement, [October] 1854, LMA/H01/ST/NC3/SU1.

33. Bermondsey Annals, 1854:226; FN to Miss Gipps, 5 December 1854, LMA/H01/ST/NC3/SU14; FN to the Council of St. John's House, 11 January 1855 and LMA/H01/ST/NC3/SU18; Selina Bracebridge to Dear Sir [Rev. C. P. Shepherd], 22 January [1855], LMA/H01/ST/NC3/SU24.

34. Lady Superintendent's Diary, 1852–54, 30 January, 6 March, 31 May 1854, LMA/H01/ST/SJ/A20/2; Register of Nurses, 1849–55, LMA/H01/ST/SJ/C3/1, 81, 95, 97, 104, 113, 122–23.

35. Elizabeth Drake to Mary Jones, 4 December 1854, LMA/H01/ST/NC3/SU13.

36. Fanny Taylor, *Eastern Hospitals and English Nurses*, 2 vols. (London: Hurst & Blackett, 1856), 1:70–71; FN to Miss Gipps, 5 December 1854, LMA/H01/ST/NC3/SU14; FN to the Council of St. John's House, 11 January 1855, ST/NC3/SU18.

37. FN Note, [May 1856], BL Add. Mss 43402 f 6; FN Reports Nos. 2 and 3, June 16 and 24 1856, BL Add. Mss 43402, ff 16–25.

38. O'Malley, *Florence Nightingale*, 246–47; Sarah Anne Terrot, *Reminiscences of Scutari Hospitals in Winter, 1854–55* (Edinburgh: Andrew Stevenson, 1898), 44–45.

39. Terrot, *Reminiscences*, 73–75; see also Robert G. Richardson, ed., *Nurse Sarah Anne: With Florence Nightingale at Scutari* (London: John Murray, 1977), 127–28. Sister Elizabeth Wheeler to a relative, cited in Thomas Jay Williams, *Priscilla Lydia Sellon: The Restorer after Three Centuries of the Religious Life in the English Church* (London: SPCK, 1950), 163–64.

40. O'Malley, *Florence Nightingale*, 260; FN to Sidney Herbert, 25 December 1854, BL Add. Ms 43393 ff 45–50; *Florence Nightingale and the Crimea 1854–55*, ed. Tim Coates (London: Stationary Office, 2000), 118–21.

41. Sue M. Goldie, ed., *Florence Nightingale: Letters from the Crimea, 1854–1856* (Manchester: Mandolin, 1997), 188–89 n. 35; FN [to Charles Bracebridge], 4 November 1855, BL Add. Mss 43397 ff 171–75.

42. FN [to Aunt Mai Smith], 19 October 1855, BL Add. Ms 45793 ff 106–9, citation on f 106; FN [to Aunt Mai Smith], 16 November 1855, Wellcome Ms 8995/75.

43. FN Note [c. 1866], BL Add. Mss 45818 f33.

44. Anne Summers, *Angels and Citizens: British Military Nurses, 1854–1914* (London: Routledge & Kegan Paul, 1988), 3–4.

45. FN to Martha Clough, 18 March 1855, Raglan Papers, Leicestershire Record Office, Leicester, U.K.; Sir Ronald Roxborough, "Miss Nightingale and Miss Clough: Letters from the Crimea," *Victorian Studies* (September 1969): 77–78.

46. Margaret Wear to Sir John Hall, 7 October 1855, BL Add. Mss 39867 ff 37–38.

47. FN to Herbert, 10 December 1854, Wellcome Ms 8994/124; Nurses Sent, FNM/H01/ST/NC8/1. In fact, Nightingale no longer had all 38 nurses because a number had already been dismissed.

48. FN to Herbert, 10 December 1854, Wellcome Ms 8994/124.

49. FN to Herbert, 18 March 1855, BL Add. Mss 43393 ff 192–203; Herbert to FN, 5 March 1855, in Stanmore, *Sidney Herbert*, 1:412–16, 372–76.

50. FN to Sidney Herbert, 15 December 1854, BL Add. Mss 43393 ff 34–40, and 28 December 1854, f 57.

51. Goldie, *Letters from the Crimea*, 54; Bostridge, *Florence Nightingale*, 242.

52. Monica E. Baly, *Florence Nightingale and the Nursing Legacy* 2nd ed. (London: Whurr, 1997), 171; Hugh Small, *Florence Nightingale: Avenging Angel* (London: Constable, 1998), 172.

53. FN to Sidney Herbert, 15 December 1854, BL Add. Mss 43393 ff 34–40, citation on f 35, and 28 December 1854, ff 57–58.

54. FN to Sidney Herbert, 25 December 1854, BL Add. Mss 43393, ff 45–50, citation on ff 45–46.

55. O'Malley, *Florence Nightingale*, 197–98, 251–52, 258, 288–89; FN to Sidney Herbert, 22 January 1855, BL Add. Mss 43393 ff 101–12.

56. E. R. Norman, *Anti-Catholicism in Victorian England* (New York: Barnes & Noble, 1968), 13–16; Chadwick, *Victorian Church*, 1:272; Paz, *Popular Anti-Catholicism*, 1–3; N. A. M. Rodger, *The Command of the Sea: A Naval History of Britain, 1649–1815* (London: W. W. Norton, 2004), 48–49, 178, 575–77.

57. Sister Mary Aloysius Doyle, "Memories of the Crimea," in Luddy, *Crimean Journals*, 43.

58. Rodger, *Command of the Sea*, 577; Norman, *Anti-Catholicism*, 18.

59. Richard J. Schiefen, "Wiseman, Nicholas Patrick Stephen," in *Oxford Dictionary of National Biography* (Oxford: Oxford University Press, 2004), http://www.oxforddnb.com/view/article/29791; Chadwick, *Victorian Church*, 1:303; Paz, *Popular Anti-Catholicism*, 5–6; Norman, *Anti-Catholicism*, 52–57.

60. Chadwick, *Victorian Church*, 1:303; Paz, *Popular Anti-Catholicism*, 5–6.

61. FN to Lefroy, 16 March 1856, BL Add. Mss 43397 ff 223–27, citation on f 226; FN to Sidney Herbert, 22 January 1855, BL Add. Mss 43393 ff 105–6.

62. FN to her family, 28 July 1855, Wellcome Ms 8995/25 f 4.

63. The Free Gift Store was a result of the publication of Sister Elizabeth Wheeler's letter in *The Times*. The paper invited people to send food and supplies to an address in London, from which they would be forwarded to the soldiers in the East. Supplies flooded in, and it took a great deal of Selina Bracebridge's time to catalog and distribute them.

64. FN [to her family?], [c. end September, October 1855], Wellcome Ms 8995/62; FN to Lady Cranworth, 22 December 1855 and 10 February 1856, BL Add. Mss 43397 f 74 and 87–88; FN to Dear sir, 30 September 1855, Nightingale Collection 1/13, Boston University Nursing Archives; Goldie, *Letters from the Crimea*, 187 n. 20.

65. FN to Sidney Herbert, 25 December 1854, BL Add. Ms 43393 f 46; FN to Sidney Herbert, 4 January 1855, BL Add. Ms 43393 f 65; Luddy, *Crimean Journals*, xxi–xxii, 138.

66. Some historians believe that Moore and Bridgeman had different agreements with the government (Goldie, *Letters from the Crimea*, 54; and Martha Vicinus and Bea Nergaard, eds., *Ever Yours, Florence Nightingale: Selected Letters* [Cambridge, Mass.: Harvard University Press, 1990], 97). In fact, Bridgeman signed essentially the same agreement with the government as Moore. It differed only in inconsequential detail (Luddy, *Crimean Journals*, xv, n. 24, 122–23).

67. Bermondsey Annals, 1854:242–43.

68. FN to Sidney Herbert, 25 December 1854, BL Add. Mss 43393 ff 45–50, citation on f 46; Bishop William Delany to Bridgeman, 8 May [1855], quoted in Doyle, "Memories of the Crimea," 44–45; Taylor, *Eastern Hospitals*, 1:5–6.

69. Vicinus and Nergaard think that Nightingale had little clinical nursing experience (*Ever Yours*, 3–4). She actually took a longer period of training, three months, at Kaiserswerth in 1851 than most ladies were taking in the London hospitals in the 1860s and 1870s, and she did much of the hands-on night nursing at Harley Street. See also Joyce Schroeder MacQueen, "Florence Nightingale's Nursing Practice," *Nursing History Review* 15 (2007): 29–49, for her clinical work after the Crimean War.

70. FN to Herbert, 25 December 1854, BL Add. Mss 43393 ff 45–50 and ff 51–56; Bridgeman, "Account of the Mission," 128–31.

71. Cook, *Florence Nightingale*, 1:77–9, 491, 502; Bostridge, *Florence Nightingale*, 119–21; Mary C. Sullivan, *The Friendship of Florence Nightingale and Mother Mary Clare Moore* (Philadelphia: University of Pennsylvania Press, 1999), 12–14.

72. Luddy, *Crimean Journals*, x–xi; Doyle, "Memories of the Crimea," 9, 50.

73. Bridgeman, "Account of the Mission," 143–47, citation on 145.

74. Bermondsey Annals, 1854:231.

75. Bridgeman, "Account of the Mission," 129; Dr. Whitty to Mary Clare Moore, 1 February 1855, Bermondsey Annals 1855:244–45.

76. FN to Uncle Sam Smith, 16 March 1856, BL Add. Mss 45792 ff 25–27.

77. Mark Harrison, "Hall, Sir John," in *Oxford Dictionary of National Biography* (Oxford: Oxford University Press, 2004), www.oxforddnb.com/view/article11974, accessed 31 July 2008; FN [to Charles Bracebridge], 4 November 1855, BL Add. Mss 43397 ff 171–75; FN [to her Aunt Mai Smith], 14 November 1855, Wellcome Ms 8995/74; FN to Col. Lefroy, 28 January 1856, Wellcome Ms 5479/4, f 4.

78. *The Times* Fund was organized by the newspaper and provided clothing and "comforts" for the men. It was separate from the Free Gift Store. Its commissioner, Mr. Mac-Donald, worked closely and amicably with Nightingale.

79. Herbert to Lord Raglan, 24 December 1854, in Stanmore, *Sidney Herbert*, 1:369; Goldie, *Letters from the Crimea*, 4–8.

80. FN [to Aunt Mai Smith], [October 1855], BL Add. Mss 45793 ff 106–09, citation on f 107; FN [to Charles Bracebridge], 4 November 1855, BL Add. Mss 43397 ff 171–75; FN [to her family], 14 November 1855, Wellcome Ms 8995/74.

81. FN to the War Office (hereafter WO), 1 and 5 March 1855, 2 April 1855, 1555656 ff 1–6, citation on f 1, WO, National Archives, U.K.; FN to Elizabeth Herbert, 2 April 1855, BL Add. Mss 43396 ff 27–9; FN to Sir Benjamin Hawes, 2 April 1855, 155656/66 ff 1–6, citation on f 1, WO, National Archives, U.K.

82. Goldie, *Letters from the Crimea*, 156–57; Bridgeman to Rev. S. Woollett, 2 September 1855, BL Add. Mss 39867 ff 28–29; FN to Hall, 14 July 1855, BL Add. Mss 39867 ff 17–19; FN to Hall, 21 September 1855, BL Add. Mss 39867 ff 31–32.

83. Wear to Hall, 24 September, 7 October, and 8 and 9 November 1855, BL Add. Mss 39867 ff 34, 37–38, 59, 63; David Fitzgerald to Hall, 3 April 1856, BL Add. Mss 39867 f 107.

84. Goldie, *Letters from the Crimea*, 243–44, 192, 298–304.

85. Bridgeman to FN, 2 October 1855, cited in Bridgeman, "Account of the Mission," 185; Bermondsey Annals, 1855:266–67; FN to Hall, 15 October 1855, BL Add. Mss 39867 ff 44–46.

86. FN [to Charles Bracebridge], 4 November 1855, BL Add. Mss 43397 ff 171–75, citations on f 175.

87. Bridgeman, "Account of the Mission," 195; FN to Hall, 15 October 1855, BL Add. Mss 39867 ff 44–46.

88. Goldie, *Letters from the Crimea*, 162.

89. FN [to Aunt Mai Smith], 3 November 1855, Wellcome Ms 8995/69, ff 1–7, citation on f 4; Hall to Nightingale, 20 July and 7 November 1855, BL Add. Mss 39867 ff 20–21, 58; FN to Hall, 27 and 31 March 1856, BL Add. Mss 39867 ff 101–3; FN to Uncle Sam Smith, 3 March 1856, BL Add. Mss 45792 f 13.

90. FN [to Aunt Mai Smith], [c. October–November 1855], Wellcome Ms 8995/45; FN to Lefroy, 11 January 1856, BL Add. Mss 43397 f 213.

91. FN to Wear, 27 November and 14 December 1855; Wear to Hall, 21 December 1855; Hall to Wear, 23 December 1855, BL Add. Mss 39867 ff 73–76.

92. Bermondsey Annals, 1855:291–92.

93. Winfried Baumgart, *The Crimean War, 1853–56* (London: Arnold, 1999), 143; Vicinus and Nergard, *Ever Yours*, 98, 119–20, 131–32, 141; Goldie, *Letters from the Crimea*, 98, 128, 135–37, 156–63, 235–41.

94. Gillian Gill, *Nightingales: The Extraordinary Upbringing and Curious Life of Miss Florence Nightingale* (New York: Ballantine, 2004), 400–401, 405–10, citation on 400.

95. Cook, *Florence Nightingale*, 1:292–93; Bridgeman, "Account of the Mission," 222.

96. FN to Lefroy, 16 March 1856, BL Add. Ms 43397 ff 223–27, citations on f 225.

97. Bridgeman, "Account of the Mission," 223.

98. FN [to Aunt Mai Smith], 25 March 1856, Wellcome Ms 8996/34; FN to Mother Mary Clare Moore, 28 March 1856, Wellcome Ms 8996/37, f 3; Sister Joseph Croke, "Diary of Sister M. Joseph Croke," in Luddy, *Crimean Journals*, 77, 81.

99. Bridgeman, "Account of the Mission," 229–30.

100. FN to Lefroy, 5 April 1856, BL Add. Ms 43397 ff 228–30, citations on f 230.

101. Confidential Report on the Nursing System, Since Its Introduction to the Crimea on the 23rd January 1855, National Archives, U.K., War Office 43/963, cited in Goldie, *Letters from the Crimea*, 298–302; FN to Lefroy, 11 January 1856, BL Add. Mss 43397 ff 205–16, citations on ff 208, 206, 209.

102. FN to Herbert, 21 February 1856, BL Add. Mss 43393 ff 215–17; Stanmore, *Sidney Herbert*, 1:13, 16–17, 91–94; 2:444–45.

103. Citations here and in the next three paragraphs are from Herbert to Nightingale, March 1856, in Stanmore, *Sidney Herbert*, 1:417–19.

104. FN to Sidney Herbert, 3 April 1856, Wellcome Ms 8996/42 ff 1–3, citation on f 1.

105. Cook, *Florence Nightingale*, 1:343–45.

106. Bostridge, *Florence Nightingale*, xx–xxii.

107. Hall to Bridgeman, 28 March 1856; Bridgeman, "Account of the Mission," 225; Bostridge, *Florence Nightingale*, 296.

108. FN, Notes, [July–August 1856], BL Add. Mss 43402 ff 159–61, citation on f 161; FN to Elizabeth Herbert, 17 November 1855, BL Add. Mss 43396 ff 40–5, citation on f 43.

109. FN, Notes, [July–August 1856], BL Add. Mss 43402 ff 159–61, citation on f 160.

110. The five Bermondsey nuns were so successful that Nightingale requested three more. They arrived in November 1855. Nurses Sent, 32, FNM/H01/ST/NC8/1.

111. Luddy, *Crimean Journals*, xiii–xiv; Bridgeman, "Account of the Mission," 223, 246.

112. Bostridge, *Florence Nightingale*, 256.

113. FN, Notes, [July–August 1856], BL Add. Mss 43402 ff 159–61, citation on f 160.

3. The Dream of Nursing the Empire

1. Judith Godden, *Lucy Osburn, a Lady Displaced: Florence Nightingale's Envoy to Australia* (Sydney: Sydney University Press, 2006); Carol Helmstadter, "Reforming Hospital Nursing: The Experiences of Maria Machin," *Nursing Inquiry* 13, no. 4 (2006): 249–58; Judith Godden and Carol Helmstadter, "Women's Mission and Professional Knowledge: Nightingale Nursing in Colonial Australia and Canada," *Social History of Medicine* 17, no. 2 (2004): 157–74.

2. Monica Baly, *Florence Nightingale and the Nursing Legacy*, 2nd ed. (Philadelphia: BainBridgeBooks, 1997), 9; "metropolitan" was later dropped.

3. For example, Florence Nightingale (hereafter FN), draft letter [1853], Wellcome Library Claydon copy (hereafter Wellcome) Ms 8994/89 f 12.

4. Baly, *Nightingale and the Nursing Legacy*, 11.

5. Sioban Nelson, *Say Little, Do Much: Nursing, Nuns, and Hospitals in the Nineteenth Century* (Philadelphia: University of Pennsylvania Press, 2001).

6. Baly, *Nightingale and the Nursing Legacy*, 15.

7. Mary C. Sullivan, *The Friendship of Florence Nightingale and Mary Clare* (Philadelphia: University of Pennsylvania Press, 1999); Carol Helmstadter, "The First Training School for Nurses," *History of Nursing Journal* 4, no. 6 (1992–93): 295–309, and 5, no. 1 (1994–95): 3–18.

8. Judith Godden, "Victorian Influences on the Development of a Professional Identity within Nursing," in *Scholarship in the Discipline of Nursing*, ed. G. Gray and R. Pratt (Melbourne: Churchill Livingstone, 1995), 239–54.

9. Baly, *Nightingale and the Nursing Legacy*, 27.

10. Hugh Small, *Florence Nightingale: Avenging Angel* (London: Constable, 1998).

11. Sue Goldie, ed., *"I have done my duty": Florence Nightingale in the Crimean War* (Manchester: Manchester University Press, 1987), 288.

12. Small, *Nightingale: Avenging Angel*, 88.

13. Patricia Jallard, *Death in the Victorian Family* (Oxford: Oxford University Press, 1996), chap. 1.

14. Nightingale Fund, *The Nightingale Fund* (London: Nightingale Fund, 1862), 3, and *Statements Exhibiting the Voluntary Contributions Received by Miss Nightingale* (London, 1857), 33, London Metropolitan Archives (hereafter LMA), HO1/ST/NC/18/02/001 and HO1/ST/NC/18/02/003. Conversions to current values can only be imprecise, but the purchasing power of the fund in 1860 was roughly equivalent to £3,108,082 (US$5,014,930) in 2008. Lawrence Officer, "Purchasing Power of British Pounds from 1264 to Present," MeasuringWorth, 2008, http://www.measuringworth.com/ppoweruk; Lawrence H. Officer and Samuel H. Williamson, "Computing 'Real Value' over Time with a Conversion between U.K. Pounds and U.S. Dollars, 1830 to Present," MeasuringWorth, 2009, http://www.measuringworth.com/exchange. Thanks to David Godden for his assistance with this issue.

15. FN to Haldane Turriff and sent to Lucy Osburn [hereafter Osburn], 22 April [1869], British Library Additional Manuscripts (hereafter BL Add. Mss) 47757 f 107.

16. FN to Elizabeth Torrance, 24 June 1870 and 25 December 1870, Sydney Hospital (thanks to donor Hilary Davidson).

17. For example, FN to William Mayne, 19 September 1866, in *New South Wales Legislative Assembly: Votes and Proceedings*, 1866, 41; FN to Henry Parkes, 24 October 1866, Mitchell Library, Sydney MS C362, reel 1465.

18. D. A. B. Young, "Florence Nightingale's Fever," *British Medical Journal* 311 (1995): 1697–1700.

19. For example, FN to [Sir Harry Verney], fragment c. 1869, Wellcome Ms 9003 f 135.

20. Cf. Mark Bostridge, *Florence Nightingale: The Woman and Her Legend* (London: Viking, 2008), 331.

21. Amanda Foreman, *Georgiana, Duchess of Devonshire* (London: HarperCollins, 1998), 158.

22. Jharna Gourlay, *Florence Nightingale and the Health of the Raj* (Burlington, Va.: Ashgate, 2003); Gérard Vallée, ed., *Florence Nightingale on Health in India*, in *Collected Works of Florence Nightingale*, ed. Lynn McDonald, vol. 9 (Waterloo, Ont.: Wilfrid Laurier University Press, 2006), and *Florence Nightingale on Social Change in India*, in *Collected Works of Florence Nightingale*, ed. Lynn McDonald, vol. 10 (Waterloo, Ont.: Wilfrid Laurier University Press, 2007).

23. Florence Nightingale, *Cassandra and Other Selections from Suggestions for Thought*, ed. Mary Poovey (New York: New York University Press, 1992).

24. Baly, *Nightingale and the Nursing Legacy*, chap. 2.

25. Robert Dingwall, Anne Marie Rafferty, and Charles Webster, *An Introduction to the Social History of Nursing* (London: Routledge, 1988), 51.

26. Baly, *Nightingale and the Nursing Legacy*, 32.

27. Ibid., 35.

28. FN to Henry Bonham Carter [hereafter Bonham Carter], 19 December 1867, BL Add. Mss 47715 f 140.

29. Roy Wake, *The Nightingale Training School, 1860–1996* (London: Haggerston Press/Nightingale Fellowship, 1998); Dingwall et al., *Social History of Nursing*, chap. 4; Godden, *Lucy Osburn*, chap. 6.

30. Baly, *Nightingale and the Nursing Legacy*, 42.

31. Godden and Helmstadter, "Women's Mission and Professional Knowledge"; Carol Helmstadter, "Early Nursing Reform: A Doctor-Driven Phenomenon," *Medical History* 46 (2002): 325–50.

32. Godden, *Lucy Osburn*, chap. 6.

33. FN to Torrance, 24 June 1870.

34. Godden and Helmstadter, "Women's Mission and Professional Knowledge," 163–64.

35. Henry Parkes to FN, 21 July 1866, BL Add. Mss 47757 ff 1–2.

36. Alison Bashford, "Medicine, Gender, and Empire," in *Gender and Empire*, ed. Philippa Levine (Oxford: Oxford University Press, 2004), 112–33.

37. *The Cambridge Social History of Britain, 1750–1950*, 3 vols., ed. F. M. L. Thompson (Cambridge: Cambridge University Press, 1990), 2:15.

38. Bonham Carter to FN, 8 August 1868, BL Add. Mss 47716 ff 3–4.

39. Harriet Dowling to Nightingale, 23 January, 11 February, 17 June, and 13 November 1863, BL Add. Mss 57757 ff 152–59.

40. Florence Nightingale, "Note on the Aboriginal Races in Australia," *Transactions of the National Association for the Promotion of Social Science* (1864): 552–58.

41. Maria Rye to FN, 20 May 1865, BL Add. Mss 47757 ff 163–66; FN to Lord Shaftesbury [December 1865], BL Add. Mss 45799 f 183, and [c. 10 December 1865], f 192.

42. FN to Colonists of South Australia, 28 January 1858, Wellcome Ms 8997 f 62.

43. Gourlay, *Nightingale and the Health of the Raj*, 72.

44. Sarah Wardroper to FN, 12 October 1866, BL Add. Mss 47729 f 33; FN to Parkes, 24 October 1866.

45. Nightingale Probationers Record, Book A, LMA/HI/ST/NTS/C4/1. Note that there are numerous errors in the list by Monica Baly published in several places, including Baly, *Nightingale and the Nursing Legacy*, appendix 3.

46. Sarah Wardroper to FN, 19 June 1867, BL Add. Mss 47729 f 300.

47. Godden, *Lucy Osburn*, chaps. 4 and 5.

48. Osburn to FN, 27 March 1868, BL Add. Mss 47757 ff 71–73.

49. Godden, *Lucy Osburn*, chap. 7.

50. Ibid., 132.

51. Ibid., chap. 14.

52. Osburn to Bonham Carter, 2 June 1868, LMA/HOI/ST/NC/18/009/001.

53. FN to Bonham Carter, 2 December 1867, BL Add. Mss 47715 f 126.

54. Anne Marie Rafferty, *The Politics of Nursing Knowledge* (London: Routledge, 1996).

55. *God Bless you, My Dear Miss Nightingale: Letters from Emmy Carolina Rappe to Florence Nightingale*, ed. Bertil Johansson (Stockholm: Bertil Johansson, 1977), 7, 33–34; FN to Bonham Carter, 4 June 1867, BL Add. Mss 47714 f 204.

56. Osburn to FN, 9 October 1868, BL Add. Mss 47757 ff 88–89.

57. John Sutherland to FN, 25 July [1868], BL Add. Mss 45753 ff 51–53.

58. FN to Bonham Carter, 24 November 1871, BL Add. Mss 47717 f 12.

59. FN to John Sutherland, 2 December 1868, BL Add. Mss 45753 f 119.

60. FN to Bonham Carter, 19 December 1871, BL Add. Mss 47717 ff 9, 21.

61. Ibid., throughout 1873, BL Add. Mss 47717 and BL Add. Mss 44718.

62. Ibid., 29 November 1872, BL Add. Mss 47717 ff 120–21.

63. Leonore Davidoff, *The Best Circles: Society, Etiquette and the Season* (London: Cressett Library, 1986), 80.

64. Osburn to FN, 3 September 1873, BL Add. Mss 47757 f 147.

65. Godden, *Lucy Osburn*; Judith Godden, "'Like a Possession of the Devil': The Diffusion of Nightingale Nursing and Anglo-Australian Relations," *International History of Nursing Journal* 7 (2001): 52–58.

66. Godden, "Like a Possession of the Devil."

67. Baly, *Nightingale and the Nursing Legacy*, 151–52.

68. Wake, *Nightingale Training School*, 251.

69. Helmstadter, "Reforming Hospital Nursing."

70. Nightingale Probationers Record Book, Book B, 1871–78, LMA/HI/ST/NTS/C4/2, entry 65.

71. FN to Maria Machin (hereafter Machin), 25 July 1875 and 4 May 1876, Nightingale Papers, Thomas Fisher Rare Book Library, University of Toronto, Toronto, Canada. All subsequent references to Nightingale's letters to Machin are also from Fisher Library.

72. Machin to FN, 18 April 1873, BL Add. Mss 47745 ff 4–5, and 26 May 1874, ff 21–22.

73. Nightingale Probationers Record Book, Book B, entry 65. Agnes Jones was one of the first "lady probationers" and became lady superintendent of the Liverpool Work-house Infirmary. After she died in 1868, Nightingale sought to recruit similar nurses by eulogizing her.

74. The classic study of passionate heterosexual female friendships is Carroll Smith-Rosenberg, "The Female World of Love and Ritual: Relations between Women in Nineteenth-Century America," *Signs* 1, no. 1 (1975): 1–29.

75. FN to Machin, 21 August 1873.

76. Ibid.

77. Nightingale Probationers Record Book, Book B, entry 65.

78. FN to Machin, 7 November 1877.

79. *Gazette,* 9 November 1877, clipping in LMA/HI/ST/NC15/34/3.

80. FN to Machin, 26 August 1874.

81. Charles Brydges, letter, 1 November 1877, *Gazette* clipping in LMA/HI/ST/NC15/34/28; FN to Machin, 14 April and 1 May 1875.

82. FN to Machin, 5 April 1876.

83. Ibid., 5 April and 21 May 1876.

84. Judith Godden and Carol Helmstadter, "Conflict and Costs when Reforming Nurs-ing: The Introduction of Nightingale Nursing in Australia and Canada," *Journal of Clinical Nursing* 18, no. 19 (2009): 2692–99.

85. Godden and Helmstadter, "Women's Mission and Professional Knowledge."

86. FN to Machin, 5 April 1876.

87. FN to Bonham Carter, 23 March 1874, BL Add. Mss 47718 f 9.

88. FN to Machin, inscription in book, 12 August 1874.

89. FN to Machin, 4 May 1876.

90. Ibid., 22 October 1877.

91. Ibid., 7 November 1877.

92. Ibid., 13 December 1877.

93. Ibid., 2 May 1878.

94. Ibid., 7 September 1878 and 19 February 1879.

95. Ibid., 21 August 1878.

4. Rhetoric and Reality in America

1. Susan Reverby, *Ordered to Care: The Dilemma of American Nursing, 1850–1945* (New York: Cambridge University Press, 1987), 16–21.

2. Ann Preston, *Nursing the Sick and the Training of Nurses* (Philadelphia: King and Baird, 1863).

3. Barbra Mann Wall, *Unlikely Entrepreneurs: Catholic Sisters and the Hospital Market-place, 1865–1925* (Columbus: Ohio State University Press, 2005).

4. Joan Lynaugh, "Nursing in Philadelphia," *American Association for the History of Nursing Bulletin* (Spring 1988): 1–4.

5. Jowett Papers at Balliol, f 61 (Benjamin Jowett's notes on conversations with Flor-ence Nightingale). I am grateful to my colleague Carol Helmstadter for this reference.

6. Florence Nightingale, *Notes on Nursing: What It Is and What It Is Not,* 1st U.S. ed. (New York: D. Appleton, 1860).

7. Mary Clymer's diaries can be found at the Barbara Bates Center for the Study of the History of Nursing, University of Pennsylvania, Philadelphia.

8. Karen Buhler-Wilkerson, *No Place Like Home: A History of Nursing and Home Care in the United States* (Baltimore: Johns Hopkins University Press, 2001).

9. Ibid., 21.

10. *The Times,* 14 April 1876.

11. The physician Osler was renowned for reforming medical education though clinical teaching. See Kenneth M. Ludmerer, *Learning to Heal: The Development of American Medical Education* (New York: Basic Books, 1985), 66–67 and 250–51.

12. Nancy Tomes, *The Gospel of Germs: Men, Women and the Microbe in American Life* (Cambridge, Mass.: Harvard University Press, 1998).

13. Charles E. Rosenberg, "Florence Nightingale on Contagion: The Hospital as Moral Universe," in *Healing and History: Essays for George Rosen,* ed. Charles E. Rosenberg, 116–36 (Kent, U.K.: Wm Dawson and Sons, 1979).

14. Ibid., 124.

15. Mark Bostridge, *Florence Nightingale: The Making of an Icon* (New York: Farrar, Straus and Giroux, 2008), 335.

16. Anne Marie Rafferty, *The Politics of Nursing Knowledge* (London: Routledge, 1996), 46.

17. *New York Times,* 15 August 1910.

18. http://www.countryjoe.com/nightingale/nutting.htm.

19. Ibid.

5. Mythologizing and De-mythologizing

1. Monica Baly, "The Nightingale Nurses: The Myth and the Reality," in *Nursing History: The State of the Art,* ed. Christopher Maggs (London: Croom Helm, 1985), 43; F. B. Smith, *Florence Nightingale: Reputation and Power* (London: Croom Helm, 1982).

2. On errors in the secondary literature, and especially F. B. Smith's, see Lynn McDonald, "Florence Nightingale Revealed in Her Own Writings," *Times Literary Supplement,* 6 December 2000, 14–15; Appendix B, "The Rise and Fall of Florence Nightingale's Reputation," in *Florence Nightingale: An Introduction to Her Life and Family,* ed. McDonald (Waterloo, Ont.: Wilfrid Laurier University Press, 2001), 843–47; and "Secondary Sources on Nightingale and Women," in *Florence Nightingale on Women, Medicine, Midwifery and Prostitution* ed. Lynn McDonald (Waterloo, Ont.: Wilfrid Laurier University Press, 2005), 1039–49.

3. E. T. Cook, *The Life of Florence Nightingale,* 2 vols. (London: Macmillan, 1913); Anne Summers, *Angels and Citizens: British Women as Military Nurses, 1854–1914* (London: Routledge & Kegan Paul, 1988), 302 n. 1.

4. Hugh Small, *Florence Nightingale: Avenging Angel* (London: Constable, 1998), 3.

5. Irene Schuessler Poplin, review Small, *Florence Nightingale: Avenging Angel, Nursing History Review* 9 (2001): 235–37.

6. Richard Brooks, "Nightingale's Nursing 'Helped Kill Soldiers,'" *Sunday Times,* 8 July 2001, 14.

7. Stuart Wavell, "The Liability with a Lamp," *Sunday Times,* 1 June 2008.

8. Clive Ponting, *The Crimean War: The Truth behind the Myth* (London: Chatto & Windus, 2004).

9. Ibid., 199.

10. Florence Nightingale, *Notes on Matters Affecting the Health, Efficiency and Hospital Administration of the British Army Founded Chiefly on the Experience of the Late War* (London: Harrison, 1858) (hereafter *Matters Affecting*).

11. Keith Williams, "Reappraising Florence Nightingale," *British Medical Journal* 337 (2008): a2889.

12. Nightingale, *Matters Affecting,* 53. These points are described in detail in Lynn McDonald, *Florence Nightingale and the Crimean War* (Waterloo, Ont.: Wilfrid Laurier University Press, forthcoming).

13. Nightingale, *Matters Affecting*, 53–54.

14. Williams, "Reappraising Florence Nightingale," 2.

15. Nightingale, *Matters Affecting*, preface to section II, ix.

16. Ibid., preface to section III, x.

17. Copy of a letter from Nightingale to John McNeill, 24 October [1856], Wellcome Trust (hereafter Wellcome) Ms 8997/9.

18. Letter, 24 February 1857, Geheimes Staatsarchiv, Berlin, f 164–65.

19. Letter to Haldane Turriff, 22 April 1869, British Library Additional Manuscripts (hereafter BL Add. Mss) 47757 f 107.

20. Richard Shannon, "An Icon and Her Intrigues," *Times Literary Supplement*, 28 May 1982, 571–73.

21. Cheryl Cordery, "Another Victorian Legacy: Florence Nightingale, Miasmic Theory and Nursing Practice," in *New Countries and Old Medicine*, ed. Linda Bryder and Derek A. Dow (Auckland, New Zealand: Auckland Medical History Society, 1995), 299.

22. Robert Dingwall, Anne Marie Rafferty, and Charles Webster, eds., *An Introduction to the Social History of Nursing* (London: Routledge, 1991 [1988]), 37.

23. Sandra Holton, "Feminine Authority and Social Order: Florence Nightingale's Conception of Nursing and Health Care," *Social Analysis*, special issue no. 15 (August 1984): 64.

24. Charles Rosenberg, introduction to *Florence Nightingale on Hospital Reform* (New York: Garland, 1989).

25. Charles Rosenberg, "Florence Nightingale on Contagion: The Hospital as Moral Universe," in *Healing and History: Essays for George Rosen*, ed. Rosenberg (New York: Science History, 1979), 125.

26. Joseph Lister, "On the Antiseptic Principle in the Practice of Surgery," *Lancet*, 21 September 1867, 353–56.

27. Monica E. Baly, "The Nightingale Nurses and Hospital Architecture," *Bulletin of History of Nursing* 11 (1986): 2.

28. *Remarks of the Barrack and Hospital Improvement Commission on a Report by Dr. Leith on the General Sanitary Condition of the Bombay Army*, adopted 6 January 1865, in *Florence Nightingale on Health in India*, ed. Gérard Vallée (Waterloo, Ont.: Wilfrid Laurier University Press, 2006), 410.

29. John Croft, *Notes of Lectures at St. Thomas's Hospital* (London: Blades, East & Blades, 1873), chap. 19.

30. "Letter to the Joint Secretaries of the Poona Sarvajanik Sabha," ed. Gerard Vallée, *Nightingale on Social Change in India*, (Waterloo, Ont.: Wilfrid Laurier University Press, 2007), 363.

31. Henry Acland to Florence Nightingale, 29 December 1895, Bodleian Library Ms Acland d70.

32. Smith, *Nightingale: Reputation and Power*, 156.

33. Ibid., 178.

34. Shannon, "An Icon and Her Intrigues."

35. Lynn McDonald, ed., *Florence Nightingale and the Nightingale School* (Waterloo, Ont.: Wilfrid Laurier University Press, 2009), appendix B, 899–900.

36. From Richard Quain, *Dictionary of Medicine* (1883), 12:749, in McDonald, *Nightingale and the Nightingale School*.

37. Quain, 12:747.

38. Ibid., 748.

39. Ibid.

40. Ibid.

41. Ibid., 742.

42. Ibid., 749.

43. Ibid., 493.

44. Ibid.

45. Note from a meeting, 19 December 1896, BL Add. Mss 47764 f 173.

46. Quain, 12:735 (see n. 35), and "Hospitals," in *Chambers's Encyclopaedia: A Dictionary of Universal Knowledge,* new ed. (London: William & Robert Chambers, 1892).

47. Nightingale, *Introductory Notes on Lying-in Institutions,* in McDonald, *Nightingale on Women,* 392.

48. Florence Nightingale to Rose Adams, 9 December 1892, Wellcome Ms 5483/57.

49. Note on a letter, 10 December 1895, BL Add. Mss 47726 f 276.

50. Monica Baly, "The Nightingale Nurses: The Myth and the Reality," in *Nursing History: The State of the Art,* ed. Christopher Maggs (London: Croom Helm, 1985), 43.

51. Probationers' registers, London Metropolitan Archives (hereafter LMA), H1/ST/NTS/C4/2–7 and H1/ST/NTS/C1/1–3.

52. "Memorandum Respecting the Admission of Gentlewomen under the Regulations for Special Probationers" (LMA/H1/ST/NTS/C27).

53. Lucy Seymer, *Florence Nightingale's Nurses: The Nightingale Training School, 1860–1960* (London: Pitman Medical, 1960).

54. Baly, "Nightingale Nurses," 34.

55. Monica Baly, "Shattering the Nightingale Myth," *Nursing Times,* 11 June 1986, 16–18.

56. Monica Baly, *Florence Nightingale and the Nursing Legacy,* 2nd ed. (London: Croom Helm, 1986), 220.

57. Smith, *Nightingale: Reputation and Power,* 173.

58. Ibid., 175.

59. Note from a meeting with F. E. Spencer, 22 January 1873, BL Add. Mss 47751 f 55.

60. Monica Baly, *Nursing and Social Change* (London: Heinemann, 1973), 64.

61. Monica E. Baly, "The Influence of the Nightingale Fund (1855 to 1914) on the Development of Nursing" (Ph.D. dissertation, University College, London, 1984).

62. Baly, *Nightingale and the Nursing Legacy,* 224.

63. Monica Baly, *Nursing and Social Change,* 3rd ed. (London: Heinemann, 1995), 119.

64. Baly, *Nightingale and the Nursing Legacy,* 220.

65. Baly, *Nursing and Social Change,* 2nd ed., 122.

66. Monica E. Baly and H. C. G. Matthew, "Nightingale, Florence (1820–1910)," in *Oxford Dictionary of National Biography* (Oxford: Oxford University Press, 2004), 40:911.

67. Dingwall, Rafferty, and Webster, "Making the Myths," in *Social History of Nursing,* 36.

68. Ibid., 37.

69. Florence Nightingale to Edwin Chadwick, 1866, cited in *Florence Nightingale on Public Health Care,* ed. Lynn McDonald (Waterloo, Ont.: Wilfrid Laurier University Press, 2004), 347–48.

70. Dingwall et al., *Social History of Nursing,* 40.

71. See Lynn McDonald, "Evidence-Based Health Care," *Evidence-Based Nursing* 4, no. 3 (2001): 68–69.

72. Richard Stone, "Florence Nightingale and Hospital Reform," in *Some British Empiricists in the Social Sciences, 1650–1900* (Cambridge: Cambridge University Press and Raffaele Mattioli Foundation, 1997), 303–37.

6. The Passionate Statistician

1. On the Nightingale family and its social, religious, and political milieu, see Gillian Gill, *Nightingales: Florence and Her Family* (London: Hodder and Stoughton, 2004).

2. Mark Bostridge, *Florence Nightingale: The Woman and Her Legend* (London: Viking, 2008), 170.

3. Ibid.

4. M. Eileen Magnello, "Victorian Vital and Mathematical Statistics," *BSHM Bulletin: Journal of the British Society for the History of Mathematics* 21, no. 3 (2006): 219–29.

5. Karl Pearson, *The Life, Letters and Labours of Francis Galton,* vol. 2 (Cambridge: Cambridge University Press, 1924), 250.

6. John Eyler, *Victorian Social Medicine: The Ideas and Methods of William Farr* (Baltimore: Johns Hopkins University Press, 1979), 161.

7. Pearson, *Francis Galton,* 250.

8. Ibid., 414–15.

9. Egon Pearson, ed., *The History of Statistics in the 17th and 18th Centuries, Against the Changing Background of Intellectual, Scientific Thought: Lectures by Karl Pearson, 1923* (London: Griffin Pub, 1975), 74.

10. Lytton Strachey, *Eminent Victorians: Cardinal Manning, Florence Nightingale, Dr. Arnold and General Gordon* (London: Chatto & Windus, 1918), 117.

11. F. B. Smith, *Florence Nightingale: Reputation and Power* (London: Croom Helm, 1982), 12.

12. Florence Nightingale, *Notes on Matters Affecting Health, Efficiency, and Hospital Administration of the British Army: Founded Chiefly on the Experience of the Late War* (London: Harrison, 1858).

13. Florence Nightingale, *Notes on Hospitals* (3rd ed.: 1862) (London: Longman, Roberts and Green, 1859); Florence Nightingale, *Introductory Notes on Lying-in Institutions* (London: Longman, Green, 1871).

14. Eyler, *Victorian Social Medicine,* 160–61.

15. Zachary Cope, *Florence Nightingale and the Doctors* (London: Museum Press, 1958), 299.

16. Ibid., 99–100.

17. See Eyler, *Victorian Social Medicine,* 167–68.

18. See replication of the graph in I. Bernard Cohen, "Florence Nightingale," *Scientific American* (March 1984): 250.

19. William Farr to Florence Nightingale, 16 November 1858, cited in Eyler, *Victorian Social Medicine,* 121.

20. Ibid.

21. Monica Baly and H. C. G. Matthew, "Nightingale, Florence (1820–1910)," *Oxford Dictionary of National Biography* (Oxford: Oxford University Press, 2004), http://www.oxforddnb.com/view/article/35241). Also see Monica Baly, *Florence Nightingale and the Nursing Legacy,* 2nd ed. (London: Whurr, 1997).

22. Florence Nightingale, *Hospital Statistics and Hospital Plans, Reprinted from the Transactions of the National Association for the Promotion of Science* (London: Emily Faithfull, 1862; reprint, London: Victoria Press, 1981).

23. "Proceedings of the Statistical Society from 20th November 1860 to 16th June, 1863," *Journal of the Statistical Society of London* 26 (1863): 445–50. See William Farr, "Miss Nightingale's 'Notes on Hospitals,'" *Medical Times and Gazette,* 13 February 1864, 166–67.

24. Cope, *Nightingale and the Doctors,* 104.

25. Florence Nightingale to Benjamin Jowett, 3 January 1891, cited in *Dear Miss Nightingale: A Selection of Benjamin Jowett's Letters,* ed. E. V. Quinn and J. M. Prese (Oxford: Clarendon Press, 1987), 423–24. Also cited in Sir Edward Cook, *The Life of Florence Nightingale,* vol. 2 (London: Macmillan, 1913), 396.

26. Although Nightingale was aware of the statistical innovations of Francis Galton in the mid-1870s, her statistical ideas were more directly aligned with those of Adolphe Quetelet and especially William Farr, both of whom were well established and renowned by the time she began to pursue her interest in statistics. As a medically trained statistician, Farr and his statistical innovations, especially his mortality rates, bore the most direct relevance to Nightingale's work. Galton was two years younger than Nightingale and thus not as well established as Quetelet and Farr in the 1850s. Moreover, Galton's

emphasis on statistical variation, rather than statistical averages, and his interest in heredity and eugenics did not impinge directly on Nightingale's work.

27. Pearson, *Francis Galton*, 419–20.

28. Ibid., 416.

7. An Icon and Iconoclast for Today

1. Department of Health, *Modern Matrons—Improving the Patient Experience* (London: Department of Health Publications, 2003), 3–5.

2. Florence Nightingale, *Notes on Hospitals*, 3rd ed. (London: Longman, Roberts and Green, 1863).

3. Sarah Waller and Hedley Finn, *Enhancing the Healing Environment: A Guide for NHS Trusts* (London: King's Fund, 2004).

4. Florence Nightingale, *Notes on Nursing* (Stroud: Tempus Publishing, 2006 [1859]).

5. Florence Nightingale, "Letter to Her Nurses, 1872," in Nightingale, *Florence Nightingale to Her Nurses: A Selection from Miss Nightingale's Address to Probationers and Nurses of the Nightingale School at St. Thomas' Hospital*, ed. Rosalind Nightingale Nash (London: Macmillan, 1914), 10.

6. Florence Nightingale, "Sick-Nursing and Health-Nursing," in *Women's Mission: A Series of Congress Papers on the Philanthropic Work of Women*, ed. Angela Georgina Burdett-Coutts (New York: Scribner, 1893), 186.

7. Debbie Singh, *Policy Brief: How Can Chronic Disease Management Programmes Operate across Care Settings and Providers?* (Copenhagen: World Health Organization, 2008).

8. Nightingale, "Sick-Nursing and Health-Nursing," 190.

9. "Letter to her Nurses, 1897," cited by Barbara Montgomery Dossey, Louise Selanders, Deva-Marie Beck, and Alex Attewell, *Florence Nightingale Today: Healing, Leadership, Global Action* (Silver Spring, Md: American Nurses Association, 2005), 296.

10. Department of Health, *Transforming Community Services: Enabling New Patterns of Provision* (London: Department of Health, 2009).

11. Nightingale, "Sick-Nursing and Health-Nursing," 189, 191, and 197.

12. P. Griffiths, A. Renz, J. Hughes, and A. M. Rafferty, "Impact of Organisation and Management Factors on Infection Control in Hospitals: A Scoping Review," *Journal of Hospital Infection* 73, no. 1 (2009): 1–14.

13. Healthcare Commission, *Investigation into Outbreaks of Clostridium difficile at Maidstone and Tunbridge Wells NHS Trust* (London: Healthcare Commission, 2007); Healthcare Commission, *Investigation into Mid Staffordshire NHS Foundation Trust* (London: Healthcare Commission, 2009).

14. Healthcare Commission, *Investigation into Mid Staffordshire*.

15. "Soldiers Face Neglect, Frustration at Army's Top Medical Facility," *Washington Post*, 18 February 2007; "Walter Reed and Beyond: A Washington Post Investigation," www.washingtonpost.com/wp-srv/nation/water-reed/index.html (accessed 19 October 2009); "The 2008 Pulitzer Prize Winners: Public Service," www.Pulitzer.org/citation/2008-Public-Service.

16. NHS Institute for Innovation and Improvement, "The Productive Series," http://www.institute.nhs.uk/quality_and_value/productivity_series/the_productive_series.html (accessed 18 August 2009).

17. Nightingale, *Notes on Nursing*, 42–43.

18. Linda H. Aiken, Sean P. Clarke, Douglas M. Sloane, Julie Sochalski, and Jeffrey H. Silber, "Hospital Nurse Staffing and Patient Mortality, Nurse Burnout, and Job Dissatisfaction," *Journal of the American Medical Association* 288, no. 16 (2002): 1987–93; Anne Marie Rafferty, Sean P. Clarke, James Coles, Jane Ball, Philip James, Martin McKee, and Linda H. Aiken, "Outcomes of Variation in Hospital Nurse Staffing in English

Hospitals: Cross-Sectional Analysis of Survey Data and Discharge Records," *International Journal of Nursing Studies* 44, no. 2 (2007): 175–82; Anne Marie Rafferty and Sean Clarke, "Editorial: Nursing Workforce; A Special Issue," *International Journal of Nursing Studies* 46, no. 7 (2009): 875–78; Sean P. Clarke and Nancy E. Donaldson, "Nurse Staffing and Patient Care Quality and Safety," in *Patient Safety and Quality: An Evidence-Based Handbook for Nurses,* ed. Rhonda G. Hughes, Publication No. 08-0043 (Rockville, Md.: Agency for Healthcare Research and Quality, 2008), http://www.ahrq.gov/qual/nurseshdbk/docs/ClarkeS.pdf (accessed 19 August 2009).

19. Peter Griffiths, Simon Jones, Jill Maben, and Trevor Murrells, *State of the Art Metrics for Nursing: A Rapid Appraisal* (London: King's College London, National Nursing Research Unit, 2008); Jill Maben and Peter Griffiths, *Nurses in Society: Starting the Debate* (London: King's College London, National Nursing Research Unit, 2008); Department of Health, *Framing the Nursing and Midwifery Contribution: Driving Up the Quality of Care* (London: Department of Health, 2008).

20. Maben and Griffiths, *Nurses in Society.*

21. Sue Machell, Pippa Gough, and Katy Steward, *From Ward to Board: Identifying Good Practice in the Business of Caring* (London: King's Fund, 2009).

22. Maben and Griffiths, *Nurses in Society.*

23. Royal College of Nursing, *Breaking Down Barriers, Driving Up Standards: The Role of the Ward Sister and Charge Nurse* (London: Royal College of Nursing, 2009).

24. Nightingale, *Notes on Nursing.*

25. Cited by Dossey et al., *Florence Nightingale Today,* 278.

26. Nightingale, *Notes on Hospitals,* preface.

27. Florence Nightingale, "Letter to Her Nurses, 1876," cited in Dossey et al., *Florence Nightingale Today.*

28. Nightingale, *Notes on Hospitals,* 13–14.

29. Nightingale, "Sick-Nursing and Health-Nursing," 187 and 194–96.

30. Ibid., 184–205.

31. Elizabeth Barry, "Celebrity, Cultural Production and Public Life," *International Journal of Cultural Studies* 11 (2008): 251.

CONTRIBUTORS

JUDITH GODDEN is a professional historian and Honorary Associate with the Department of History, University of Sydney. She was previously a faculty member both at the School of Public Health and the Faculty of Nursing and Midwifery at the University of Sydney. Her book, *Lucy Osburn, a Lady Displaced: Florence Nightingale's Envoy to Australia* (Sydney University Press, 2006), was short-listed for Australia's 2008 National Biography Award. She is currently completing a biography of the twentieth-century Australian nurse Gwen Burbidge, to be published by the College of Nursing (NSW) and, with Carol Helmstadter and Joyce MacQueen, a book on nursing reforms in London teaching hospitals 1800–1860.

CAROL HELMSTADTER is a registered nurse and graduate of Wellesley College and Columbia University. Over the course of her career she was actively engaged in professional issues, spending seven years as a union representative and president of an eight-hundred-member Ontario Nurses Association (ONA) Local and then seven years as ONA's Government Relations Officer. Now retired, she is an accomplished independent scholar. She is the recipient of the Centennial Nursing Award from the Canadian Nurses' Association and the Lavinia L. Dock Award from the American Association of the History of Nursing. She is best known for her work on nineteenth-century nursing at the London teaching hospitals.

JOAN E. LYNAUGH is Professor Emerita of Nursing at the University of Pennsylvania, where she held the History of Nursing and Health Care Term Professorship. She is Director Emerita of the Barbara Bates Center for Nursing History and former Associate Dean and Director of Graduate Studies at the University of Pennsylvania School of Nursing. Dr. Lynaugh's honors include the Centennial Nursing Heritage Award from the American Nurses Association, the Lavinia L. Dock Award, the Hannah Lectureship of the Canadian Association for the History of Nursing, the Agnes Dillon Randolph Award from the University of Virginia, and the Distinguished Alumni Award from the University of Rochester.

M. EILEEN MAGNELLO is a Research Associate in the Department of Science and Technology Studies at University College London. She is a graduate of La Roche College, Pittsburgh; received a Master's degree in statistics from Kent State University, Kent, Ohio; and received a PhD in modern history (history of science) from St. Antony's College, Oxford University. She is a trained statistician and is well known for her extensive publications on the history of science and technology and on the life and statistical innovations of the Victorian statistician Karl Pearson.

LYNN MCDONALD is University Professor Emerita, University of Guelph, Ontario, Canada. She is the editor of the *Collected Works of Florence Nightingale,* a sixteen-volume project published by Wilfred Laurier University Press, Waterloo, Canada, now in its fourteenth volume. She has been writing about Nightingale and other women theorists since her 1993 book, *Early Origins of the Social Sciences.* McDonald is also a public health advocate. As a member of the Canadian Parliament, she succeeded in getting the Non-smokers' Health Act adopted in 1988. She has been a women's advocate (first "Ms." in the House of Commons), and was president of the Canadian National Action Committee on the Status of Women. She has an honorary doctorate from York University, Ontario.

SIOBAN NELSON is Dean and Professor at the Lawrence S. Bloomberg Faculty of Nursing at the University of Toronto, Canada. She is a registered nurse and graduate in history from La Trobe University, Melbourne, earned a PhD in humanities from Griffith University, Brisbane, Australia, and completed postdoctoral studies in health sciences and history at the University of Melbourne. She has written in the areas of history, professional issues, health policy, and the organization of practice. She is editor-in-chief of the scholarly journal *Nursing Inquiry*. She is also coeditor, with Suzanne Gordon, of the series The Culture and Politics of Health Care Work for Cornell University Press. Her recent award-winning work, *The Complexities of Care: Nursing Reconsidered*, was coedited with Suzanne Gordon.

ANNE MARIE RAFFERTY is Dean of the Florence Nightingale School of Nursing and Midwifery, King's College, London, a position she has held since 2004. She received a bachelor's degree in nursing studies from Edinburgh University and a Ph.D. in modern history from Oxford University. She won a Harkness Fellowship to study at the University of Pennsylvania, Philadelphia, and worked with Dr. Linda Aiken on the role of nursing in the Clinton health reform agenda. She was appointed Director, Centre for Policy in Nursing Research at the London School of Hygiene and Tropical Medicine, in 1994 and subsequently Head, Health Services Research Unit. Her research areas include the health-care workforce, health sector reform and patient outcomes, nursing history, and policy analysis.

ROSEMARY WALL is a postdoctoral Research Associate at the Florence Nightingale School of Nursing and Midwifery, King's College, London, where she is researching the history of British colonial nursing. She received a bachelor's degree in economic and social history from the University of Liverpool and a master's degree in the history of science, medicine, and technology from Imperial College, London, and she completed a doctoral dissertation on the use of bacteriology in England from 1880 to 1939, also at Imperial College. This work was followed by a postdoctoral position researching the history of late colonial medicine in Kenya at Oxford University.

INDEX

Note: Italic page numbers refer to tables and figures.